# Thyroid C

# Overcoming Fear and Finding Fulfilment

By Dr Tom Cawood
Hospital Specialist Endocrinologist and Physician
Ph.D., M.B.Ch.B.(Hons), B.Sc.(Hons), M.R.C.P.(UK),
F.R.A.C.P.(NZ).

Copyright 2015 Tom Cawood
This book is copyright. Except for the purpose of fair review, no part may be stored or transmitted in any form or by any means, electronic or mechanical, including recording or storage in any information retrieval system, without permission in writing from the publishers. No reproduction may be made, whether by photocopying or by any other means, unless a licence has been obtained from the publisher or its agent.

*"May you live all the days of your life."*

Jonathan Swift (1667-1745)

# Contents

Foreword ............................................................................ 7

Chapter 1 - Beginning to live better with thyroid cancer ........................................................................................... 13

Chapter 2 - Finding a thyroid lump ............................. 21

Chapter 3 - Your first appointment ............................. 29

Chapter 4 - Fine Needle Aspiration ............................. 39

Chapter 5 - FNA showing thyroid cancer – what next? .53

Chapter 6 - Thyroid surgery ........................................ 65

Chapter 7 - Should I have radioiodine? ...................... 73

Chapter 8 - Taking radioiodine. .................................. 93

Chapter 9 - Follow-up; life with thyroid cancer and how to start making it better ............................................ 103

Chapter 10 - When things aren't going so well .......... 117

Chapter 11 - Living better with thyroid cancer .......... 125

Chapter 12 - Medullary thyroid cancer ...................... 135

Chapter 13 - Anaplastic thyroid cancer ...................... 145

Chapter 14 - Thyroid hormone replacement in thyroid cancer ........................................................................ 151

Chapter 15 - Closing thoughts ................................... 161

Thanks ....................................................................... 165

# Foreword

If you or someone close to you has just found a neck lump, it might be thyroid cancer. How do you feel? What lies ahead? How will you cope? How will your family cope? What next? What if...?

I'm a hospital doctor who specializes in endocrinology and general medicine, and I care for people with thyroid problems. In fact, I've spent most of the last 10 years focusing on thyroid diseases. My Ph.D. research degree looked at thyroid eye disease and my current clinical work includes thyroid out-patient clinics and dedicated thyroid cancer clinics.

Then my own bombshell. At forty years of age I was found to have a form of congenital heart disease that had severely damaged my heart and was now a potentially fatal diagnosis. I lay on the hospital bed prior to open-heart surgery with my previous hopes of how my life would likely play-out totally shattered. If I survived, life would never be like it was.

From this unusual perspective of being both a doctor and someone trying to cope with a frightening diagnosis, I have gained huge insight into the emotional devastation that thyroid cancer patients can face when dealing with this life-changing diagnosis. And that's even before they start navigating the medical system. Crucially, a thyroid cancer diagnosis will most likely force you to confront some of the bigger questions in life. Up until now you may have conveniently avoided them (I certainly had!).

Having lived through such an experience, I initially found it to be hugely unpleasant. However, having also been able to emerge out of it (with help) to live a much more fulfilling and positive existence, I have written this to try to help make the experience for others be less painful than mine. This book is a practical and emotional support that will help you get through and beyond your diagnosis of thyroid cancer. It aims to provide comfort and calm, knowledge and wisdom, and help you and your family live a better life.

A potentially life-changing medical diagnosis almost never comes at a good time. It might appear out of the blue, like being hit by a car that didn't stop at a red light. It might be the last straw that breaks the camel's back. In amongst all the confusing, overwhelming medical information, what help is offered to deal with all the rest of it? How do I cope with the possibility of not living long enough to care for my children, not seeing them grow up or get married? How do I deal with my own mortality?

Current medical systems, no matter how good they may be where you live, largely fail to address the bigger questions that arise. They are usually busy trying to get you the best possible medical outcome within difficult time constraints. But to differing degrees, we all need help with these bigger things – mortality, happiness, family, the meaning of it all. Given that you have read this far, you may also be searching for some help. Whilst this book cannot possibly divine the meaning of life, it aims to offer some practical steps to help you deal with your diagnosis, to navigate through the medical system and make some sense of it all. It also aims to encourage you to go on to live a more fulfilling and positive life in whatever time remains, than you ever did before.

I have found that knowing that my life is fragile, and possibly much shorter than I had previously hoped, has given me appreciation of how precious, unlikely and special life really is. I have been offered the liberation to live every heart beat in the best way possible, and I intend to accept that offer, for as long as I can!

If you are looking for a detailed medical textbook on thyroid cancer you should probably look elsewhere. If you really want to know the false negative rate of fine needle aspiration or the significance of BRAF gene mutations you should probably ask your specialist. However, if you are looking for the important stuff in easy-to-understand language then this book may be for you. In addition if you need help converting the medical information into something that makes sense in your life and helps you deal with the emotional consequences of thyroid cancer, then this book is for you.

A number of thyroid cancer patients kindly agreed to be interviewed for this book. I've quoted their own words throughout the book in the hope that sharing their experiences helps provide comfort and insight from those who have gone through the sort of challenges that you are facing right now.

Although probably hard to believe right now, you may look back on this time as one of the most important and ultimately positive things that could ever have happened to you.

Dr Tom Cawood, 2015

*"Wisdom comes from experience.
Experience is often a result of lack of wisdom."*

Terry Pratchett

# Chapter 1 - Beginning to live better with thyroid cancer

At first glance the suggestion that life could be better with thyroid cancer compared to life without it might sound odd. Life was good before. You might have never had to worry about your health before. You were carefree and bullet proof. If you'd given it even a passing thought, you may have thought you were going to live forever, or at least been comforted by the fact that anything different was so far off that it wasn't worth thinking about.

You may have had the normal worries, like money, your job, relationships, your latest diet, your childrens' education, your daughter's dodgy boyfriend, etc. But these probably seem much less important since your future has been threatened by the possibility of thyroid cancer.

We all have problems, and some are more important than others. While at any one time the burden of these problems can appear overwhelming, there is for many people, a recognizable priority hierarchy of these problems. Once the hierarchy has been identified it can make them much more manageable. Thyroid cancer can be looked at as an opportunity to put other problems into perspective, and help not only deal with the thyroid cancer, but to deal with the other problems as well.

An unavoidable reality for us all is that we have only a finite amount of time living on this earth. A set number of heart beats. Getting the most out of life is partly about not wasting too many of those heart beats. Getting the most out of every moment of every day.

Most of us seek happiness and fulfillment in life. For each of us the precise way we might wish to achieve this will vary, but there are common themes that are associated with having full and happy lives. Many of them might appear like they are no-brainers: having lots of money, not having a miserable job (perhaps not having any job and winning the lottery), having a nice house, decent car, etc.

However, for many of us these things are not practically attainable and more importantly, they don't usually lead to true happiness. Most of the above examples are related to material wealth, and many have been found to be more likely to cause unhappiness – just think of the family squabbles over money, or of lonely rich people. Whilst it is true that poverty can be associated with depression and poor outcomes including poor healthy, the opposite isn't true (i.e. wealth does not equate to happiness).

**Factors linked with happiness**

There are a number of things that have been linked to happiness and fulfillment. Whilst the quality of evidence supporting them, and the importance of each factor varies hugely, some of the more common factors involved are:

1) Spending time on, valuing, and nurturing relationships and friendships.

2) Good physical and mental health.

3) Having a reasonable standard of living and satisfactory work.

4) Being able to perceive beauty in art and nature.

5) Having some form of Spirituality, Faith or Religiosity.

6) Having goals such as commitment to family and friends or social involvement rather than focusing on career success or wealth.

7) Having a relatively narrow gap between expectations and reality.

8) Setting, working towards, and achieving specific goals.

So what has all this got to do with the here and now of the possibility of having thyroid cancer? Well, part of dealing with thyroid cancer involves an appreciation of what is likely to make us happy. This is especially important if your thyroid cancer might take away some heartbeats from the total you had previously hoped for.

For the relatively lucky majority, for whom thyroid cancer is not going to reduce their total number of heart beats, then thyroid cancer can be viewed as a wake-up call that enables the person to get the most out of life. The preciousness of life and time has been forced into focus. For those with thyroid cancer that is more extensive and more likely to reduce the person's total number of heart beats, then it's arguably all the more important to take steps to value and maximize the happiness and fulfillment from what time remains.

So what can someone with thyroid cancer, even advanced thyroid cancer, actually do to live a better life from here on?

*Before my thyroid cancer I used to be worried about what I thought were big things, but now I see they were small things. These little things used to easily upset me.*

*After my diagnosis, once I knew that my life may be short, that life is precious, I kind of do my best. I now do volunteer jobs at the citizen's advice bureau; I help out at my children's school. I enjoy my time now. I don't know why I didn't do these things before. My quality of life is better. I'm lucky because my health is better than I first thought it would be – I get no symptoms from my thyroid cancer, I can live normally, and so I have more time that I first thought I would have, so not only do I live a better life, but I have time to live it. I actually feel healthier than before, physically and spiritually.*

### Suggestions of some things to work on

You may already know what to do in order to live in a more fulfilled way. You may have known it for a long time, and thyroid cancer is the catalyst for you to take those actions. If that's you, excellent go for it, do it now. If you are not so clear, here are some pointers. This can't be the complete solution for everyone, it's just a beginning.

1) Try to control what you can control, and accept what you can't
    a. Don't ruminate; if you do have worries/issues that can't be controlled or accepted, schedule 20mins worry time per day, and try to convert that time into concrete action plans.
    b. Have pen and paper by your bed, so if at night you find yourself ruminating, or your head spinning, just right down the headings and deal with them in the light of day. If the thought re-appears during the night, you can nip it in the bud, knowing that it's already on paper and so an action plan has been

       activated and so there's no need to give it any more brain time that night.
   c. Don't waste time worrying over the little stuff.

2) Acceptance of mortality (sounds simple but it can be very, very hard – there is more on this in Chapter 10).

3) Mindfulness – appreciating the now; doing the things that you value, saying 'yes' when your kids ask you to spend time with them.

4) Value those close to you.

5) Set realistic goals, and take steps to achieve them.

6) Maximize free time, including 'me' time.

7) Make a bucket list (and add an item each time you tick one off).

8) Consider taking regular exercise and eating a sensible diet.

The above is only a beginner's guide, intended to offer a few initial pointers to help you get through today, knowing that tomorrow may not be as bad as it might appear. If you are at the beginning of possible thyroid cancer then the next few months may be a rollercoaster. The following few chapters will give you an idea of what the medical steps will be over the coming months. However the process of trying to live a better, more fulfilling life, is an on-going process and I'd suggest investing as much time and effort into that transition as you possibly can. It may be one of the most important things you ever do.

*"The best preparation for tomorrow is doing your best today"*

H. Jackson Brown, Jr, P.S. I Love you.

## Chapter 2 - Finding a thyroid lump

Most thyroid cancer initially shows itself by the appearance of a lump in the neck. You might have seen it in the mirror or felt something when you swallow. You might have felt it whilst putting on a necklace or necktie. Sometimes it's someone else who notices it. These lumps are also often found when a medical scan is done for some other reason, and the thyroid lump is an incidental finding which then prompts more tests.

***I remember the moment I was looking in the mirror putting my make up on, and seeing the lump in my neck. There was clearly something going on. I didn't think cancer. Not then. I assumed it was all going to be fine.***

However it is found, the finding of the neck lump is the beginning.

People react to this in different ways. Some immediately pick up the phone to make an appointment with their doctor, whilst those at the other extreme choose to try to ignore it, hoping it will go away. It's not unusual for people to feel some degree of unease, or even dread, but this feeling doesn't straight away lead to any action, with the distractions of day-to-day life quickly taking over again.

***I was sitting at the dinner table when my daughter said: What's that lump in your neck, Mum? I thought, what's she talking about?***

*So I go and have a look in the mirror and have a feel around, and actually there was a bit of a lump there. I'd intentionally lost some weight before then and so perhaps that's why it had become more obvious. If I hadn't gone on a diet it might not have been found when it was. I just thought it would be nothing, and my daughter was about to get married so I just put it to one side until the wedding was over. I'm good at pushing things to one side and not confronting them.*

At this point you have some choices to make, and it's best to have some information to help you make the choice that's best for you:

Firstly, there are lots of different causes of a lump in the neck. For some people the lump they have found has always been there and is just part of normal anatomy, like a part of the voice box or a salivary gland. However, if the lump is definitely new then it's probably not just normal anatomy. There are lots of lymph nodes in the neck. These are part of the immune system, the system that is busily protecting you from infection plus killing off cancerous cells. Lymph nodes are like a road-side police check point, inspecting drivers' licences and breath testing all the cars (or in the body's case, all the cells), that are passing by, and arresting those that are not clean. If you have an infection in the head or neck area, such as an ear infection, throat infection, etc, the lymph nodes that are situated on the route that drains those areas often get enlarged and sometimes a bit painful, whilst they clean the infection up. This can often cause a lump in the neck, but it usually returns to normal size sometime after the infection. Lymph nodes can also enlarge for other reasons. This includes them being swollen with cancerous cells, but in that situation they don't usually return back to normal size but instead they get bigger.

Lumps within the thyroid gland can often be distinguished from lymph nodes because the thyroid gland, and lumps within the thyroid gland, are attached to the voice box (the Adam's apple structure, in the middle of the neck, about half way down from your jaw to the base of your neck). The voice box moves up and then down when you swallow, so lumps within the thyroid gland also move up and down when you swallow. In contrast lymph nodes tend to stay still when you swallow.

Importantly, the vast majority (90-95%) of thyroid lumps are harmless. By harmless I mean benign which means non-cancerous. Occasionally benign thyroid lumps can get quite big and may even need surgical removal, but the important point is that they are not cancer.

## What is my neck lump, and what should I do?

There is a long list of rare causes of neck lumps which you don't really need to know about right now. The key points to think about are that a neck lump may be:

1) a normal finding
2) abnormal but harmless (a benign thyroid gland nodule)
3) cancerous

Your next decision is to decide what to do about it. Broadly your options are:

1) Do nothing about it
2) Do something about it, but not right now
3) Do something about it now

No-one is in your shoes but you, and there may well be lots of factors that influence your decision such as your personality type, your degree of anxiety, your degree of denial tendencies, your finances, how busy you are, what your other health issues are, etc. However, a few things that may help you decide include:

1) Those who do nothing about it will almost certainly continue to worry about it. If their lump is harmless, then that is a whole lot of unnecessary worry, and arguably life is too short and precious to waste any of it on unnecessary worry. If it is a cancerous lump then doing nothing but worry about it may lead to a worse outcome, with the disease being picked up once it is more advanced and less treatable.

2) Those who decide to do something about it are likely to have a much better outcome – either it is found to be harmless, and worry is over, or it is found to be cancerous and at least then treatment can start and future challenges can be identified and faced.

3) Those who decide to do something, but not right now may run the risk of delaying, and delaying some more, as the time is never quite right. If it wasn't important enough to do anything about at the time it was first found, there is not often a more obvious time to do something about it – time can pass and it can be weeks or months before action is taken. Those can sometimes be important weeks or months, with treatment outcomes being less good as a consequence.

The standard medical advice is that if you find a lump in your neck you should get it assessed by a doctor promptly. If you or someone close to you has found a neck lump, it makes sense to call your doctor now to make an appointment. Even if you have exceptional personal circumstances, there are not many situations where doing nothing about your neck lump is a good option.

If you have made the decision to get the lump assessed, and made the appointment, there is nothing more you should do other than try to limit any worry or anxiety you have about it. You've already taken the appropriate action, and worrying about the wide range of possible outcomes is unlikely to help. It is best to get on with enjoying life, and wait for the information that will come out of your appointment. Once it is clear what you are dealing with, and what the options are, then that is the time to make further decisions.

Importantly, once you have made the decision to seek medical attention, in most cases there is no great urgency for the assessment to happen. You don't need an appointment today or tomorrow (unless you have problems with swallowing or breathing!). Even if your lump is cancerous, most thyroid cancers are very, very slow growing, and a few weeks here or there will not make any difference to the outcome.

***I'd had a lump for a long time and just thought it was an enlarged gland or fatty blob or something. I happened to change doctors, and my new doctor thought I should get it checked out. I didn't really think it was worth doing anything about it, it was genuine lack of concern. I look back and think that was just so silly. Because there was so much breast cancer and ovarian cancer in my family, I was just so fixated that I'd get one of those cancers, it was the last things on my mind that I could get thyroid cancer. It didn't even cross my mind.***

If for some reason you cannot get medical attention (with the most likely reason being financial), then the option of doing nothing now, but deciding to do something later if the lump doesn't go away, is your next best option. It's often a good idea to pick a time interval, e.g. 2 weeks or 4 weeks, and agree with yourself that if it is still there, to make the call then. This gives you some time to try to get the money together, or the time off work, or to try to get over whatever barrier is stopping you from getting the care you need.

There are always exceptions to every rule, and this book can't possibly cover all possibilities. There is the occasional situation where a thyroid lump enlarges quickly, and can start interfering with swallowing or even breathing. If this occurs then you need urgent medical attention. There are situations where the thyroid gland can become inflamed and as a result can release too much thyroid hormone into the bloodstream. This can lead to symptoms of thyrotoxicosis (such as fast pulse, feeling hot and sweaty, increased anxiety, weight loss, tremor, etc.) that also needs prompt attention. Too much thyroid hormone can amplify worry, so if you find you are perhaps excessively worried and anxious about a neck lump, make sure your thyroid hormone levels are checked at the same time that your neck lump is being assessed.

**Key points:**

There are lots of causes of a neck lump
Most neck lumps are harmless, but a few are cancerous
All new neck lumps need medical assessment
Get your neck lump assessed, and then you can either stop worrying about it, or start the process of dealing with it.

*"Action may not always bring happiness; but there is no happiness without action"*

Benjamin Disraeli

## Chapter 3 - Your first appointment

**How you might feel**

Now that you have found a neck lump, and made the decision to get medical attention, you will be facing your first appointment. You probably aren't feeling great, and have a mixture of nervousness, fear and anxiety. You may not be used to being on the receiving end of medical attention and are outside of your normal comfort zone. If you are young and previously bulletproof, having an abnormal lump in your neck can be very unpleasant. Not just the lump itself but also the realization that your health may no longer be perfect can be very hard to take. If you are towards the other end of the scale, someone with lots of medical problems, having a new problem can be that last straw.

On the other hand, if you are feeling fantastic and hugely positive, reassured by the statistics that most thyroid lumps are harmless and you are sure there is almost certainly absolutely nothing to worry about then it's good that you are feeling so good. However it's just possible that your reaction is a coping mechanism, conscious or otherwise. There's nothing wrong with feeling good, but it can be more difficult to accept bad news if you haven't truly considered that bad news could be coming your way, however unlikely that may be.

**Your first appointment**

Whatever your feelings, you still have your first appointment to face. Quite whom you are seeing will depend on which country you are in, and how the health service is set up. In many countries the first port of call will be your family physician or general practitioner, in others you may be going directly to a specialist. Whomever you see, they will probably want to hear your story first. They will want to find out the history of your neck lump – when it started, how you found it, if it's causing you any symptoms, etc. They will probably also want to know about the rest of you – any other symptoms in general, your past medical history, what medications you are on, what allergies you may have, any family history, your social history (smoking, alcohol, home situation, etc.), and a range of other questions screening for other problems. They will then want to examine you, particularly your neck. They will likely also want to do some blood tests, arrange a neck scan, and organize a needle test of your neck lump.

Every doctor I know is trying to do a good job, to provide the best possible outcome for his or her patients. However, there are many doctors I know who are not working in ideal conditions. They often don't have enough time, and they may be tired, or have other commitments that demand their attention such as being on-call for emergencies, or having sick patients on the ward. Your appointment may well be interrupted by the doctor answering phone calls. Also, everyone is different, and some doctors suit certain personalities. Even if the care provided is equal, there are some doctors that you may feel more comfortable with. In addition, whilst this appointment for you may well be one of the more significant episodes in your recent life, for the doctor you could be the thirteenth person that day that he or she has seen. Whilst they are probably trying to be empathetic, it's arguably impossible for that doctor to fully understand how you are feeling and what you are going through. If the doctor was able to appreciate all those things for all their patients, they would burnout after 3 weeks and never work again. As a result there is often a gap between what you might be expecting and what the doctor can provide, and being mindful of this gap can help you get the best outcome from the appointment.

**Preparing for your first appointment**

Here are a few things that can help the first appointment go well:

1) Try to arrive a little early for your appointment.
   This might sound obvious, but make sure you allow for traffic, parking, getting lost, etc., especially if the appointment is in an unfamiliar hospital. If you are late, the doctor will likely have even less time to spend with you, and the less time you have, the more likely that something important is missed. Also, have your latest mobile phone and landline numbers handy, as if you subsequently are waiting for important results, you want the doctor to be able to contact you easily.
2) Wear clothes that allow easy examination of your neck. Tight, turtleneck collars are not ideal.
3) Turn your phone off before you enter the consultation. The more interruptions, the less time you will have, and the less you will get out of the consultation.
4) Bring someone else with you.
   It is amazing how the two sides of the same conversation can take away quite different messages. If you are emotionally charged, anxious and worried it can be hard to accurately take things in. It's even harder to take it in if some doctor bombards you with loads of information using strange medical terminology that may be difficult to understand or retain. The doctor may use a turn of phrase, or clumsy words, which you take to mean something quite different from what he or she was

meaning*. Having someone else there to help take in what is being said can be hugely helpful, and having a joint de-brief after the appointment can also be helpful to clarify the important take-home messages.

5) Bring a list of your current medication – names of tablets, doses, and how often you take them.
Saying that you take the little white pill, and a couple of little yellow ones will likely frustrate your time-pressured physician. Offering a neat list of your meds, that he/she can keep, is ideal.

6) If possible, have a list of your previous medical problems (if any).
There may be something here that is relevant to either your current lump, or what measures may need to be taken around any future surgery or other treatments you may need.

7) Prior to the appointment, ask close family members if they have had any neck or thyroid or endocrine (hormonal) problems.
Certain thyroid problems can run in families, and having some of these details to hand can be very informative.

8) Have a list of key questions. Hopefully, your doctor will cover these during the consultation, but at the end if you have a few key questions listed, you can ensure that you have the information you are looking for.

* In one of my own appointments with my hospital specialist I heard him say that because of my heart condition I should not drive a car. I was stunned, and was so busy trying to take in this message, that I could not take in what he said in the following few sentences. My wife who was with me was able to clarify that what he actually said was that in some cases patients should avoid driving karts (not cars), where drivers race round a track in beaten up vehicles, repeatedly crashing into each other. After some confusion the specialist went on to say that there was no

good reason why I should not continue to drive an ordinary car, although he said I should try to avoid crashing (no great change there, then!).

*It's good to have somebody with me. I brought my daughter, she's a nurse, and it's so much better to have her with me to make sure that between us we understand what's going on. She would support me, listen during the appointment, take some notes. We would often have a list of questions prepared before the appointment and if they hadn't been answered during the clinic, she would be able to prompt me, to make sure we got the information we needed. It was a real help.*

As part of your assessment, unless your doctor is sure that your lump is harmless, and doesn't need further investigation, he/she will want to do additional tests. This may be some form of neck scan (usually an ultrasound scan) and a needle test of your lump.

*Every person I met was good, the problem was more the joining together of the dots, the complex workings of the medical system, and how bewildering it can feel to be in the middle of it.*

It is important to mention that the medical system that you are about to have to navigate through may be a very complex organization. There may be lots of different people you come in to contact with. This includes receptionists, nursing staff, doctors, surgeons, radiographers and more. There are many more people you don't directly come in to direct contact with but are nevertheless vital components of the machinery of modern healthcare, such as typists, administration staff, radiologists, pathologists, surgical theatre nurses, etc. Despite everyone's efforts to make your journey through this system smooth and seamless, the common reality is that it is often far from perfect. This can be frustrating and annoying. These system problems just add to the difficulties at a difficult time. Reminding yourself that no-one is perfect and no system is perfect can help keep the negative effects of such experiences to a minimum.

> *My initial FNA was equivocal, so I needed to get another one done under ultrasound guidance with a pathologist present to see if they had got enough cells. But when I went for the FNA, there was no pathologist there. With the vastness of the machinery of healthcare it's not surprising that things don't always go exactly as they should. You need to be prepared for this.*

With regard to the tests that you are likely to need the ultrasound scan is similar to the scan that pregnant women get. The operator uses a hand-held probe on the skin, with a gel-type cream to make good contact between the probe and the skin. The probe sends painless sound waves through the skin which bounce off the structures under the skin, and these are picked up by the probe and with the help of a clever computer, creates an image of the anatomy on the screen. The images are often quite blurry and require an experienced operator to be able to identify what is what. They can usually identify the thyroid gland, and nearby structures such as blood vessels (carotid artery, jugular vein, etc.) and lymph nodes. Importantly the ultrasound scan cannot usually tell whether a thyroid lump or lymph node is harmless or cancerous. There are sometimes clues as to which it is, but none of these clues are reliable enough to be very useful. So whilst the ultrasound can often tell you what is there, it can't reliably tell you whether it is cancerous or not, and for that reason what is needed is a sample of the lump. This sample is normally obtained using a needle, a process called Fine Needle Aspiration (FNA).

During an ultrasound scan it is often an ultrasonographer who is performing the scan. Whilst they are able to identify and measure various structures, they usually don't have full details of your medical history and are not in a position to give you an accurate report of what they have seen. Instead the images are viewed by a radiologist (who is a doctor), and it is the radiologist who is able to give their experienced opinion as to what has been found. Therefore during the scan it is unlikely that you will get the result – instead there may be days between the scan being done and the final report being issued. This is something I have found very difficult to deal with as a patient. I really struggled during the intervening days of uncertainty and worry whilst waiting for what might be a really important verdict. This has become easier to deal with after having many scans. I try to view the scan as just an inconvenience, and pick a date a week or so later as the important date, the date when I'm actually going to receive some information from which decisions can be made.

So having had the initial appointment, and probably also had an ultrasound scan (though no results yet!), then the next step is likely to be a Fine Needle Aspiration (FNA). Whilst this is a relatively easy test to have done, the decisions about whether to have it done and what the results might mean are sometimes a bit more controversial. Hence it gets its own chapter.

*"We demand rigidly defined areas of doubt and uncertainty!"*

Douglas Adams, The Hitchhiker's Guide to the Galaxy

# Chapter 4 - Fine Needle Aspiration

Fine needle aspiration (FNA) involves inserting a thin needle into a lump and sucking up some of the cells from within that lump. The type, shape and appearance of the cells, when viewed down a microscope by an expert, can give a good idea of what the lump actually is. There are a huge number of possible causes for neck lumps. These can't all be covered in this type of book. Instead we'll focus mainly on thyroid lumps, usually called thyroid nodules.

**FNA Results**

There are a number of different possible results from an FNA of a thyroid nodule. These fall broadly into the following groups:

Group 1: Benign (harmless) - approx. 65%
Group 2: Can't be sure - approx. 30%
Group 3: Malignant (cancerous) - approx. 5%

**Group 1: Benign**

The vast majority of thyroid nodules are benign – probably more than 95%. By benign we mean harmless; not cancerous; not able to spread. These benign nodules don't usually go on to become cancerous. If they are benign they usually stay that way forever, and don't require further treatment or investigations. Some of them may gradually grow in size over time. Occasionally they can get big enough to get in the way of things, or squash things in the neck. If this is going to happen, it usually happens gradually, over many years. It can eventually result in difficulty swallowing, a hoarsening of the voice (due to damage to nerves that control the voice box that run very close to the thyroid) and sometimes can cause breathlessness. The trachea (the windpipe) is a strong tube, held open with rings of cartilage (the same material that makes your nose, and makes shark skeletons), so it's usually quite difficult for a thyroid nodule to narrow the trachea enough to cause breathlessness. However, it can sometimes happen, particularly when the whole thyroid gland is enlarged, perhaps with multiple nodules, or when the gland extends downwards below the level of your collar bones where there is a bit less space. If that does occur, then surgery is needed to remove the enlarged thyroid gland and relieve the pressure.

Thyroid nodules are very common. If you do an ultrasound scan of normal adults, you can find one or more thyroid nodules in about 50% of perfectly normal, healthy people. These are often quite small nodules (under 1cm) and haven't / won't cause any symptoms or future ill health. As mentioned previously, more than 95% of all thyroid nodules are benign. However if you have a larger thyroid nodule, that has come to attention because of symptoms or it has become big enough to feel, then the chance of it being cancerous might be thought to be higher than average. As is typical of certain thyroid problems, things are not always what you might first think. In fact the size of a thyroid nodule doesn't have much, if any, bearing on the chance of it being cancerous.

What this all means is that even before you have your FNA of your thyroid nodule, there is a very high chance (probably more than 9 in 10 chance) that it will be a harmless, benign nodule. However, due to technical and other reasons the chance of your FNA result concluding that your nodule is benign is about 65% (between 6 or 7 out of

10). This is because a certain number of FNA tests don't get enough cells to be certain of what the nodule is. This can often happen when your thyroid nodule is partly filled with fluid (called a thyroid cyst). This is like a small water balloon. The liquid inside doesn't contain many cells so sucking out the fluid often does not yield enough cells for a clear answer. In that case you need cells from the cyst wall, which can be tricky to get even with ultrasound guidance. The cyst walls can be very thin and hard to get a decent sample from.

If you do get a benign result then this is good news. You can shed most if not all, of any thyroid nodule-related worries. You can look forward to a discussion with your doctor about what, if any, follow-up is required. In some centres they will advise to forget all about it unless it gets significantly bigger. In other centres they may want to do follow-up ultrasound and sometimes a repeat FNA. This difference in approach is because no-one knows exactly what the best thing to do is. The more thorough the follow-up plan, the less likely it is that something important will be missed and only picked up later. On the other hand if a person gets lots of investigations, this may increase their worry and result in unnecessary treatment. It's a balancing act. The fact that only a very, very small number of people with initial benign FNA of a straight-forward nodule will be found to have thyroid cancer in the future is obviously a good thing, but that makes it a bit harder to know whether and how to follow such people up. Part of that balance is that in some countries having a delayed diagnosis of thyroid cancer can have medico-legal consequences for the doctor involved, perhaps resulting in a more thorough follow-up strategy. A somewhat delayed diagnosis of thyroid cancer often has very little, if any, influence on the eventual outcome. The majority of thyroid cancer is very slow-growing, and is cured or controlled over the long term. This makes it more difficult to balance the risk of harm versus risk of benefit from the various follow-up plans.

In a nutshell, a benign thyroid nodule is a really good result. It's worth having a discussion with your doctor about whether any follow-up is needed, and if so what that follow-up might be. There are pros and cons of the various follow-up plans. The chance of future thyroid problems is very small. Whether you are someone who likes to have regular health checks, or whether you prefer to only deal with problems if and when they occur, can influence what the best strategy is for you.

From a broader perspective, it might be helpful for you to consider all the various things that concern or worry you. Maybe write them down in a list. Then cut them out and try to arrange them in order of priority. Perhaps get your partner or friend to help you arrange them. Are you able to place a rough figure on how likely it is that the item you have listed will happen? (e.g. old age, versus plane crash, versus losing your job, etc.).

If you have a benign thyroid nodule, and you have listed that on your worry list, I'd suggest the chance of that ever causing you serious ill health is very small. If you never have routine follow-up, and forget all about it, and only get it further investigated if it gets significantly bigger or causes more symptoms, the chance of this strategy causing you serious harm is tiny. It would be way less than 1%, probably less than 1 in 1000. The benefit from regular follow-up is unknown, but if the risk of harm is less than 1 in 100, and my educated guess is that it is less than 1 in 1000, then there would need to be 100 to 1000 people having regular follow-up for 1 person to benefit. What are the chances of that person being you? (1 in 100 to 1 in 1000 – i.e. very unlikely). Yet you are certain to be harmed in some ways (repeated appointments, possible financial costs, worry re results, etc.) if you do have regular follow-up.

I can't tell you what's right for you, but when I list my worries in order of priority, with the chance of these things actually happening, a benign thyroid nodule would not feature, and if it did it would be right at the bottom of my list, alongside being hit by a meteor or spontaneously combusting. Everyone is different and if your benign thyroid nodule is on your worry list, then that's fine. It may mean that relatively speaking, you don't have much in the way of other worries if a genuinely low-risk possibility is on your list. There are some people however whose list contains things that are extremely unlikely to happen, yet omit things that are either much more likely, or arguably much more important. If you look at factors that are known to be associated with happiness and fulfillment (such as those listed in Chapter 1), then focusing on these things may be more likely to help you achieve a better quality of life.

Another useful strategy is to identify those things that appear on your worry radar that are either very unlikely (such as harm arising from not having follow-up of a benign thyroid nodule, plane crash, winning the lottery, etc.) and/or are quite outside of your control (meteor strike, global financial markets), and place them all in the same physical or metaphorical bucket. You then actively promise yourself that you will refuse to waste valuable heartbeats worrying about anything that belongs in this bucket. You've already decided to address these issues by determining that no significant good can come from worrying about such things, they have been placed in the bucket, where they will remain. They are not un-dealt with, they have just been considered, and considered to be worthy only of the bucket, and that action in itself makes their worry value evaporate. With time you can learn to quickly recognize that whenever one of these things blips on your radar, you can visualize it being placed in the bucket, where it will remain, quiet, calm and dealt-with. This frees up time and space for you to focus on the things that do need to be actioned, which hopefully includes things that are more likely to bring you happiness and fulfillment.

Having digressed a bit from benign thyroid nodules, let's move on to the other FNA result groups: 2 (can't be sure), and group 3 (cancerous)

**Group 2: Can't be sure**

Not all FNA results can give a definite answer. Sometimes there are not enough thyroid cells obtained, and the pathologist can't offer a reliable diagnosis. "Insufficient for diagnosis" is the usual comment, and often a repeat FNA is advised. This doesn't mean that it is cancerous, or that it is not cancerous, it just means they can't tell and need another sample containing more cells before they can offer an opinion. This can often be the case if a thyroid nodule is made up largely of fluid (the nodule is often referred to as cystic), because although the nodule may decrease in size after it's been drained of some of the fluid, there often aren't many cells in the fluid, and so the FNA doesn't give a clear answer. The pathologist really needs cells from the cyst wall before they can determine whether the nodule is benign or not.

A second group of nodules falls in this 'not sure' group. These are the follicular neoplasms. With this group, even though there may be lots of cells in the FNA sample, the pathologist is still left 'not sure' because these nodules can only be labeled benign or malignant once the whole nodule has been removed. This allows the whole architecture of the nodule, including the edges of the nodule to be looked at to see if there are signs of the cells spreading outside the nodule. Most of these follicular neoplasms are benign (roughly 70%), but the other 30% turn out to be malignant. This 30% number is too big for most of us to be comfortable with, which is why if your FNA result shows a follicular neoplasm, your doctor will likely advise that you have at least that half of your thyroid gland surgically removed. Then, the pathologist can have a good look at the whole nodule down the microscope and tell how it has been behaving. If, as in the majority, it is behaving like a benign, non-invading nodule, it then gets called a benign follicular adenoma. With this result nothing more needs to be done. You are left with the other half of your thyroid which is usually enough to make sufficient thyroid hormone so that you don't need thyroid hormone replacement tablets. If, however, the pathologist sees that it was behaving in a malignant, invading way, then it gets labeled as a follicular thyroid cancer. In this case it is usually best to have the other half of the thyroid removed (in a second operation at a later date). This means you won't have enough thyroid gland left, and you will need thyroid hormone replacement, but the surgery may well have removed all of your thyroid cancer. This second operation to remove the remaining half of the thyroid gland (the completion thyroidectomy) allows for the possibility of you having radioiodine treatment as part of your package of care, if that is thought to be of benefit for you (there's more about radioiodine in Chapters 7 & 8).

There are a number of other FNA findings that may also fall into this 'not sure' group. There are a variety of names for them, depending on the wording and interpretation that your local pathologists have. Things like 'atypia of uncertain significance', and other names, which all basically mean 'not sure'. In this setting your doctor and you should discuss what it might mean, and whether it's wise to sit tight, and watch and wait, or be more proactive, perhaps with a repeat FNA (perhaps with ultrasound guidance), or even surgery. There's a fair amount of judgment calls here, with no single right answer for everyone and it often pays to talk the options through to help weigh up the pros and cons. The right option for you may not be the right option for everyone else (compare what might be best for someone of 23 years of age who wants to start a family, to that of someone who is 85 years of age, with bad heart trouble and a recent stroke who really wants to attend their granddaughter's wedding next month). With the guidance of your care team, you should be able to find a path that works for you, which hopefully leads you to a more definite 'benign' or 'cancerous' diagnosis, which in turn allows the way forward to become clear.

## Group 3: Malignant (cancerous)

If you are reading this book because you have, or fear you may have, thyroid cancer then you may have jumped straight to this bit. That's fine. Let's get on and deal with it. Once you know what you are dealing with, the right path of action becomes clearer, and things can be broken down into smaller manageable stages that can be tackled one step at a time. Good information can help the whole experience become less frightening, less overwhelming, and allow you to get on with overcoming each hurdle.

Cancerous means the same as malignant. Cancer begins with a big C, and for some people is inherently more upsetting so many people use 'malignant' instead. It all means something that is growing in an uncontrolled manner. However, there is a huge range of extremes. Just like the behavior of children, who can range from being so close to well-behaved that it's extremely difficult to tell if they are anything other than angelic, to the other extreme of a wild child, kicking and screaming at all he sees, so thyroid cancers can also display a wide range of behavior. Many thyroid cancers are so close to being well behaved, that they will never go on to cause significant harm. They may very slowly spread to adjacent structures (typically lymph nodes in the neck), but even once there, they sit there, doing nothing but growing very, very slowly, over decades, and will never cause any trouble. At the other extreme there are some thyroid cancers that are aggressive, that spread far and wide, and do cause trouble. These rarer thyroid cancer situations can end up causing significant symptoms and can be life-limiting.

***Understanding what cancer means is so important. Most people think that cancer equals death. I wish someone had explained to me that all cancer means is that cells are not growing in a controlled way, and what's important is where the cells are, how they behave and how they can be treated and controlled. If I'd had a very simple explanation of what I'd got, that would have been so valuable.***

Most of the cancer diagnoses from thyroid nodule FNA will be types of thyroid cancer. For a very small number your FNA may have shown a non-thyroid cancer, such as a lymphoma, or a cancer from elsewhere in the body. These are outside the scope of this book, and need to be discussed with your doctor, as the range of possible outcomes is hugely broad. We will concentrate on cancers of the thyroid gland.

There are a variety of different types of thyroid cancer and we'll go on to deal with these in turn in the coming chapters. There are even subsets of different types of cancer within these groups, but much of this detail is not important now. The key things are 1) that you have had it diagnosed and 2) now there is a clear path forwards.

Whilst it is hard to grasp the range of likely outcomes when the word 'Cancer' has been mentioned, there are 2 broad ideas that may be helpful to consider now.

1) Thyroid cancers, in general, are at the more well behaved spectrum of cancers. You may be familiar with common cancers such as breast, lung and colon cancer. These are obviously potentially devastating diseases. Whilst their treatment is continuously improving, a broad principle remains that if these cancers have spread from the site of initial growth, the outlook is likely to be poorer, with the disease quite likely to be life-limiting despite all the best treatment that modern science has to offer. Therefore in these types of cancers there is a pressure to get the diagnosis and the treatment quickly, to get things dealt with before the cancer has spread.

However, with thyroid cancer things are often quite different. Even if thyroid cancer is spread outside of the thyroid, it is still often possible to cure the disease, or at least keep it in check, so that it does not cause significant symptoms or any shortening of life. This is partly because of the generally slow-growing, well-behaved nature of many thyroid cancers, but also due to the effective treatments that are available (such as surgery and radioiodine). In this setting there is less pressure. There is less need to be certain that every thyroid nodule is not malignant, less pressure to rush into treatment, less pressure to have radioiodine today rather than next month, less pressure in general. The outcome of most thyroid cancers is relatively good, even if it has spread. And whilst these generalizations may not be overly helpful for you (they may not apply to your particular cancer, and even if they do you may not believe them until the next 40 years have passed and you have long out-lived your initial thyroid specialist) they do paint a relatively positive backdrop against which you can view your disease and your future.

2) In the setting of thyroid cancer, from which most people do well, it provides an opportunity for you to learn the lessons that the disease provides, and it usually also provides the years within which to apply those lessons. The new perspectives and priorities that living with a potentially life-threatening disease can offer are of lesser value if you have little time left in which to do things differently. Thyroid cancer however, for many, can help you decide how to live your life for the better and also give you sufficient remaining heart beats with which to live that better life.

From where you are sitting right now, it may not look so good. Things may look bleak. Whether things are bleak, or just look to be bleak, it may now be time to tackle the practical things, one step at a time, and the next step is deciding what to do with your FNA diagnosis.

*"It may be unfair, but what happens in a few days, sometimes even a single day, can change the course of a whole lifetime..."*

Khaled Hosseini, The Kite Runner

# Chapter 5 - FNA showing thyroid cancer – what next?

*My doctor called me; he'd never called me before. As soon as I knew it was him I knew something was up.*

*I felt shocked. Even though I had a feeling that I might be in that few percent that are cancerous, when it did turn out that my FNA showed cancer, I still felt gut-wrenching shock.*

If your FNA result shows thyroid cancer you may well be in a whirl. You probably can't think straight, you may be feeling waves of emotion, perhaps even panic. You may feel sick, off your food, distracted by upsetting thoughts of what this might mean for your family, of what it might mean for you. You may well only be seeing the C of Cancer, and thinking of all the personal experiences you have had with Cancer, such as relatives, friends, things on TV. It may feel overwhelming, and awful.

*When I got my diagnosis of thyroid cancer, I think my world changed color; suddenly changed. The sun still shines, but I feel so different. I feel the world is now so strange to me. It's totally different from that moment.*

Whatever your reaction, now is the time to pause, take a few deep breaths, and take things one step at a time. One thing that may help you with this is the fact that the outcome from thyroid cancer is usually relatively good.

*It wasn't until I was talking to the specialist, who said something about stage 1, when I thought 'Oh my goodness, he's talking about thyroid cancer. That's just so weird, it's not what I expected'. Perhaps it was really naïve of me. I'm not really a worrier, and despite the lump and the FNA and the hospital appointment, I just didn't think I'd be in the small statistic of people that have thyroid cancer. I was in shock during that appointment – but very quickly I was given the statistics of 98% of people in my position doing well, and not dying from their thyroid cancer, so I went so quickly from being told about thyroid cancer to then being told about the likely good outcome, that I didn't really have to time to get worried about it.*

Remember that unlike many other types of cancer, with thyroid cancer, even if it has spread, it can often be controlled and even cured with treatment. This is partly because thyroid cancer cells are often very good at sucking up iodine, and so if patients are treated with radioactive iodine, the cancer cells suck this up too, and so end up sucking up a specific poison which kills these cells, and leaves the rest of the person pretty much untouched.

**Thyroid cancer stages and outcomes**

If you like numbers, here are some which might help. Thyroid cancers are put into 4 different categories (called stages) depending on a number of factors such as tumor size, and how widely it has spread. Stage 1 is the stage with the least advanced cancer, with the best outlook, and stage 4 is the stage with the most advanced cancer with the worst outlook. For most patients with Stage 1 or 2 thyroid cancer, the 5-year survival from the cancer is nearly 100%. Those with Stage 3 thyroid cancer have a 70 to 90% 5 year survival, and those with Stage 4 cancer have a 30 to 50% 5 year survival rate.

These numbers are based on the outcome of lots of patients, and may not apply accurately to you (you may do better or worse than these average figures), but the overall message is that with thyroid cancer, even if it has spread, there is a good chance that you will either be cured, or that the cancer will be kept under control for the long-term.

> *The big thing I've thought about a lot with my thyroid cancer, is that even though the statistics say that you're likely to have a good outcome with thyroid cancer, those figures don't necessarily apply to you. They apply on average, but not necessarily to you. So when I've dodged a bullet with my brain tumor (which was benign) I thought why should I be lucky twice? And so those numbers mean nothing to me; I didn't really believe that my thyroid cancer was going to behave like the average and go well.*

Hopefully, the knowledge of the usually good outcomes of thyroid cancer will allow you to take a few more deep breaths, make a cup of tea (or glass of wine, or whatever), and take some time to pause and calm down a little. Then when you are ready, take things one step at a time, and find out more about your particular cancer – what it is, where it's at, and what to do next.

Because there is such a wide range of possible outcomes from thyroid cancer, you need to narrow this down a bit. Thinking of all the possible outcomes in the world is too difficult, too exhausting, and arguably a waste of time and emotion. You need to know the likely range of outcomes for you, and then come to terms with understanding and accepting the worst and the best outcomes, as well as the most likely, average outcome. An important part of this is talking to your doctor, to find out the type and stage of your thyroid cancer.

*I was away for the weekend and I was drinking a glass of wine, when the phone rang. The second I hear the surgeon's voice I know the news is not good. She probably did use the word cancer, but she didn't need to. As soon as I heard her voice I knew exactly what she was ringing to tell me. If she were ever to phone me again I know I would immediately snap back to that moment.*

**Types of thyroid cancer**

Broadly speaking there are 4 types of thyroid cancer:
1) Papillary
2) Follicular
3) Medullary
4) Anaplastic

These are listed roughly in order of their behavior, with papillary being probably the least aggressive, with the best outcome, and anaplastic (which is very rare) being the most aggressive with the worst outcome. Papillary and Follicular are similar, in that they largely behave like undisciplined thyroid cells (they usually suck up radioiodine and so can be killed with radioiodine). Medullary is quite different, and is usually dealt with by surgery alone. Anaplastic is very difficult to treat, and the focus is more on managing symptoms and coping with all the issues that surround coping with an aggressive, treatment-resistant tumor.

The usual sequence of events is:

1) Find lump
2) Have FNA (with or without a thyroid ultrasound scan)
3) FNA shows cancerous, or possibly cancerous cells
4) Have surgery to remove the thyroid gland
5) Possibly have radioiodine to wipe out as many remaining thyroid cancer cells as possible
6) Long term follow-up, to identify and deal with any recurrence

Your doctor will often be able to tell you what type of thyroid cancer you have, based on your FNA results. Sometimes the FNA alone is not able to give the full answer. Either way, the next step is usually to go ahead with surgery to remove all of the thyroid gland. In some cases (those where the FNA has found follicular cells, but cannot tell whether they are cancerous or not), the best step is to remove half of the thyroid. The pathologist will then slice up the removed half of the thyroid and look at this half down the microscope. From this they can tell whether the cells are behaving in a benign, disciplined way (thyroid follicular adenoma) or in a malignant, undisciplined, cancerous way (thyroid follicular cancer). If it looks like cancer, then the remaining half of the thyroid needs to be removed in a second operation.

**Why remove the whole thyroid?**

There is usually a need to remove the whole thyroid because:

1) There may well be areas of thyroid cancer in the other lobe of the thyroid gland (particularly papillary cancers, which are often multiple, scattered throughout the thyroid).

2) It helps with accurate staging of the cancer, which in turn helps decide what the best treatment is for you.

3) It allows you to be treated with radioiodine. If large parts of your thyroid gland are left in the neck, then these healthy cells will suck up the radioiodine, so very little will be sucked up into the cancer cells. This means that any remaining cancer cells are less effectively killed off by the radioiodine. Radioiodine works best at killing thyroid cancer cells when there aren't many healthy thyroid cells left in your body.

**How to deal with where you are at now.**

At this point, you likely have had an FNA result that indicates thyroid cancer, you probably know what type it is, but have little idea how advanced (what stage) your cancer is at. Whilst you are hoping for a relatively good outcome, no-one knows for sure if this is going to be how things turn out for you. There is a large amount of uncertainty, and probably a large amount of anxiety and worry regarding how this might affect you and your family.

One of the first things to acknowledge and try to accept is that there is uncertainty. This can only be reduced once you have had surgery, and your tumor has been staged. However, even then, there will be uncertainty. Arguably there has always been uncertainty in your life, but this may be one of the first times when this uncertainty is health-related and is difficult to deal with.

*One of the first things we did when we found out it was cancer was to tell our friends at church. The Elders prayed for me, and we got huge support and comfort,*

***and I trusted that things would turn out for the best.
From that point on I didn't have any real worries.***

One of the common responses to this is to start imagining the various possible outcomes. This can be useful, but it can sometimes add to the overall levels of anxiety and distress. One tendency that can be particularly harmful is to identify the possible problem, but to stop there, and not identify the next step; i.e. the solution or outcome from that particular problem. For example, you may imagine that your cancer is not fully removed by the up-coming surgery. This naturally will be a cause of concern. The next step is after identifying this problem, to consider the solution to this problem, to see what is beyond your fear. This often dissipates much of the anxiety that was previously wrapped around that outcome.

In this case, if surgery doesn't cure it, the next stage is to imagine what would be next (such as radioiodine, on-going surveillance, and further surgery and/or repeat radioiodine if needed), mindful of the overall good survival numbers given above. Another example might be to imagine that your thyroid cancer cannot be cured, and may one day be the cause of your death. This is obviously pretty big stuff, and hard for anyone to deal with. The challenge here is to accept that one day, something will be the cause of everyone's death. We usually don't know what or when that might be, but it is an inevitability that we cannot avoid. The priorities then include acceptance (of the impermanence of everything), making the most out of every day that we have, and trying to get to the point that we can focus on the positives that are around us every day, rather than allowing the fact of our eventual passing to detract from the now.

**A tool for managing uncertainty and worry**

Different people deal with things in different ways. Some people never worry about tomorrow, and others do little else! What works for one person may not work so well for the next. There is often a grief-type reaction that people feel after a significant diagnosis, like thyroid cancer. Many people will naturally adjust, and come to terms with things over weeks or months. If you find that this is not happening, and that your thyroid cancer diagnosis is having more of a negative effect on you than it should, or more of a negative effect on you than you want, then you may benefit from expert help. However, for now, it may be enough to try to limit your imagination to the likely outcomes, try to identify the scenarios that you are most concerned about and try to think of the next steps beyond that, to help the worry fade back down to where it belongs.

*I'm a kind of glass-half-full sort of person, and I think a positive outlook is really important. Each time a clinic visit, or scan or appointment goes well, it just reminds me how blessed I have been.*

If you find that your outlook is particularly negative, one useful technique can be to perform an imagination task. Think of something you do commonly, such as a commute to work, or a visit to the supermarket. Now imagine the worst possible series of events during that common task. For example on the commute to work you have a flat tyre, you scald your private parts with your coffee, you knock down several pedestrians, get hit by a meteor, then have a swig of whisky to calm down and get arrested for drunk-driving, etc., etc. You get the picture.

Next, think of that same task but think of the best possible series of events. For example on the way to work you think of a fantastic idea to solve all your work problems plus ensure world peace, you collect the post on the way to work and find that the bank have decided to pay off your mortgage simply because you are a great person, you get a phone call on the way to work saying that you have won the lottery, then your boss calls to say that you are so great you only need to work 2 days per week, whilst driving to work you see that a meteor is about to strike, but you see it before everyone else, and quickly skid you car round to close the road so that when the meteor strikes no-one gets hurt and you later get a medal for bravery and general awesomeness. Again, you get the picture. Now, assuming that you really let your imagination rip, and were able to identify the two extremes, you can probably see that either extreme is extremely unlikely. The most likely outcome is somewhere around the middle point between these extremes. Now try to apply this same process to what you are currently feeling negative about. Try to find equally unlikely extremes of outcome, and from that try to identify the likely middle ground. Once you have visualized this middle ground, then that is the likely path to be expecting, until or unless you get hard facts that deviate you off that path, one way or another.

The next practical step is to get on with getting your thyroid cancer removed.

*The worst bit for me was the wait between my diagnosis and my surgery. If I had known that the outcome would likely be the same whether I had to wait 2 weeks or 2 months, then it would have been much easier. But when you think that with every passing day your cancer might have grown to the point where it might kill you, 2 weeks can feel like a year. If the patient knows it's going to grow very slowly, if they have this information right at the start, then it's so much easier to take.*

*"The future depends on what you do today"*

Mahatma Gandhi

## Chapter 6 - Thyroid surgery

This step is all about getting your thyroid cancer removed. This involves surgically taking out as much of the thyroid as the surgeon can. If the cancer has not spread outside of the thyroid, then cutting out the thyroid gland will usually cure the cancer. Job done. If the thyroid cancer has spread outside of the thyroid gland it usually goes to the lymph nodes in the neck, and if these are big enough to find, and safe to get at, the surgeon may well try to remove these lymph nodes too.

***I had to just hand over control to the staff and trust their professionalism, and the nurses and everybody were really good. On the day there was a bit of delay waiting for my surgery time but I just put things to one side, did my Sudoku book, and my time soon came. The most uncomfortable thing was the tight stockings they put on me afterwards!***

Not many of us relish the prospect of having surgery of any type. Thyroid surgery is neither the biggest surgery nor the smallest surgery, it's somewhere in between. It's bigger than getting a toenail done, smaller than a heart coronary bypass operation, it's somewhere in between, about the same as getting your gallbladder out. By this I mean that you will need to come in to hospital, and in most centres you'll be in hospital for 2 to 5 days. You will be up on your feet later the same day, feeling a bit tender and perhaps a bit groggy, and you will probably have a thin plastic tube draining any fluid from under the scar. Some people feel bright and ready to go really soon, whereas other might feel pretty tired for a while and need some rest.

***The day after surgery I had so many visitors, friends and family, and they were all really nice but I found it awful, I was just so, so exhausted. I really needed someone, a nurse, someone, anyone to take control and tell them that it was too much, that I just needed a rest. I really needed someone, like my husband, someone close to limit the visiting. I didn't feel able to tell people myself, I was trying to be welcoming but I was wrecked.***

The drain gets removed a day or two later, and you usually head home without the drain, and ready for some ice-cream and DVDs or a good book, to take it easy for a few days. You'll likely be able to resume your normal activities in a week or 2. If you've had your entire thyroid removed, you'll need to take thyroid hormone replacement tablets for the rest of your days. This is just a rough guide as each hospital has its own variations of how best they do the surgery and post-operative care, and it depends a bit on your type of thyroid cancer, where it is, how advanced it is, etc. Your surgeon should be willing and able to answer any specific questions you may have.

There are various information sheets available if you want more details (e.g. The Royal College of Surgeons UK, Entitled "Get Well Soon, Helping you to make a speedy recovery after a thyroidectomy; easily found via Google)

### Potential problems with thyroid surgery

As with any operation there is always the chance of an undesired outcome, and thyroid surgery is no different. For those who like to know the numbers and details, here goes:

If 20 people are going for surgical removal of their thyroid (called thyroidectomy), 19 of those people will have a smooth, uncomplicated surgery and a smooth post-surgical recovery. They'll have a horizontal scar, usually about 5 to 6 cm across, usually placed in a skin crease. An advantage of having a wrinkly neck is that such scars are usually very well hidden. The scar starts off pink and obvious, and with time gets closer to skin color, and gets thinner, and harder to see.

Of the 1 in 20 people who have some sort of problem with the surgery, the problem is usually minor such as superficial wound infection that clears with antibiotics, or some bleeding that leaves a bruise that goes away with time. Occasionally there is more significant bleeding which is why most people are kept in hospital overnight. Whilst in hospital any bleeding can be more quickly identified, and treated promptly (e.g. with simple pressure, or if need be with a return to surgery to locate the leaking blood vessel and close it off). There are 2 other possible adverse effects with thyroid surgery that are worth being prepared for:

1) Low calcium levels in the blood
This is called hypocalcaemia and this happens because there are 4 small glands that control blood calcium levels, called parathyroid glands, and these are located close to or within the thyroid. They are only about pea-size, and can be really hard to find. They are often embedded within the thyroid and so get removed when the thyroid is removed. Sometimes, even if they are found and carefully left behind, they get bruised or their blood supply gets affected, such that they don't work well. This is often temporary, but can occasionally be permanent. If these parathyroid glands aren't working well, they don't make enough parathyroid hormone, and this results in the blood calcium levels dropping. A slight drop in the calcium level causes no

symptoms, but if it drops too far then muscles and nerves can get a bit twitchy. The nerves can result in tingling sensations, particularly around the mouth. The muscles can cramp up, causing muscle spasms, which if not treated can occasionally be dangerous. Serious hypocalcaemia is very rare (less than 1 in 100 people). After your surgery you will likely be having a number of blood tests to check the calcium level, which is another reason that people are often kept in at least over night after thyroid surgery. If the calcium level is low, then that is treated with an intravenous drip of fluid containing calcium, and later vitamin D and calcium tablets. With time (days / weeks) usually the parathyroid glands recover and no on-going treatment is required. Occasionally the parathyroid glands don't recover, or all 4 of them were removed at surgery, in which case long term vitamin D and calcium tablets are required to keep the calcium level high enough to prevent symptoms, but not so high that it causes problems like kidney stones.

***My surgeon was really good. He came round twice a day and explained things. The main problem was my calcium which was a bit low, and I got tingling and needed calcium and vitamin D tablets, but it was easier to handle because I had been warned and things had been explained so well.***

2) Hoarse voice
The nerves that control the voice box run very close to the thyroid gland. One of these nerves loops right down in to the chest before coming back up to the voice box (God only knows why). These nerves may already be under pressure from the adjacent thyroid gland, and so may not be functioning at 100% prior to the operation. Often a vocal

cord check is done pre-operatively to make sure the voice box and the nerves supplying it are OK. During the operation every effort is made to identify these nerves and so avoid injuring them. However even with the most skilled surgeon it is not always possible to fully protect these nerves, especially if they are caught up with the thyroid cancer. If one of the nerves is damaged this can result in a hoarse voice. This is usually temporary, but can occasionally be permanent (less than 1 in 100 operations). This can be a major problem, particularly if public speaking or singing is important for that person, for example in their job.

*I still have some trouble with my voice. I can't sing the high notes anymore. I used to enjoy singing in a country band, and in the church choir, but I can't do it anymore. It actually hurts to try to sing. But, I mean, who cares; I'm alive! It's a small price to pay, I just enjoy listening to other people now.*

If the voice is injured during the operation things can be done to improve it, such as an injection into one of the vocal cords, but sometimes permanent hoarseness is the end result. If one of the nerves was already damaged, then your surgeon may not want to operate unless absolutely necessary because injuring the other nerve can lead to the vocal cords closing off the airway, and so require a tracheostomy (formation of a passage from the windpipe to the outside world via a hole in the skin below the voice box). This is exceedingly rare – I have never personally seen this happen.

There is sometimes a fine line between having enough information to make a reasonably informed decision, and having too much information. There are so many ways that adverse things can happen (meteor strike, shark attack, freak fall on to tarmac, car crash, random attack, choking on steak, etc.). If too much emphasis is placed on very unlikely outcomes then this can be unnecessarily paralyzing. We'd all stay at home, and even then be scared of slipping to our death in the shower. It is perhaps best to focus on what is the likely outcome, whilst being reasonably mindful of the potential for important rare outcomes. With this in mind, 19 out of 20 people who have their thyroid gland cut out will have a smooth, problem-free experience. For the 1 in 20 who have some form of problem, it is usually minor. The chance of a bad outcome from surgery is very small, and this chance is almost certainly much less than the chance of a bad outcome from NOT having the surgery.

*The hospital ward was full of old people who snored and made lots of rude noises all night so I couldn't wait to get out of there! On day 3 it was pretty sore, but again, nothing I couldn't handle. My voice was really flat initially, like a monotone, and I couldn't sing for 3 months, but from the start my voice was loud enough so I knew I'd be able to get back to work which was a big relief. As it turned out I was back in the classroom teaching just a week after the operation.*

Therefore, now that you are armed with some of the facts and will have any further questions answered by your surgeon, you are now ready for the next step – getting the surgery done. Then after surgery, if required, you'll be talking to your thyroid physician about radioiodine and then future follow-up.

*"One thing you have to realize from now on is that it doesn't matter if this is a dream or not. Survival depends on what you do, not what you think"*

Rebecca McKinsey, Anterria

# Chapter 7 - Should I have radioiodine?

Once your surgery is behind you, the next step in dealing with your thyroid cancer is to consider radioiodine treatment. Whilst this might sound scary, it sounds much worse that it is. Many other non-thyroid cancers require chemotherapy and or radiotherapy, and in comparison radioiodine is a walk in the park. Radioiodine doesn't hurt, and usually you don't feel anything. The main downside is that you will be a bit radioactive for some days afterwards. This means you may need to keep a distance from others and be careful where you pee, until your radioactivity levels drop. The thought of that is probably much worse than the reality, so let me take you through it.

**How radioiodine works**

The one thing that normal thyroid cells do really well is suck up iodine from the bloodstream, and transport the iodine to the inside of the thyroid cell. The thyroid cells' job is to manufacture thyroid hormones, and iodine is one of the raw materials for that manufacture process. On the surface of every thyroid cell is a transporter, which is like a revolving rotating door that you find in some hotels. Imagine the street is the blood stream and the pedestrians are molecules of various salts, like sodium, calcium, potassium and iodine. Imagine this particular hotel only lets skinny short people in, and so has a revolving door that is small and narrow. Everyone on the street wants to get into this hotel, because the street is hugely crowded and stinking hot, and the hotel is nicely air-conditioned and gives out free cool drinks and ice-cream. Each pedestrian that gets near to the door tries to get in, but if they are too tall or too wide they wont fit, and the pressure of the moving crowd quickly moves them on down the street. When the short skinny person (iodine) comes along, it fits in the door, and is gently ushered into the hotel lobby and so travels from the street, into the hotel. With time the lobby gets quite full of skinny short people, enjoying their ice-cream. The concentration of skinny short people per square meter becomes much higher inside the hotel than on the street. As rooms become available the short skinny people make their way further inside the hotel, leaving the lobby behind. With time they are given enough ice-cream that they turn into something different (fatter people), which is the equivalent of thyroid hormone.

Similarly, in the body, when you eat a meal the nutrients get absorbed from the gut into the circulation (and become the various different types of pedestrians and traffic). As the blood passes through the thyroid any iodine gets taken up by the thyroid cells whilst most other molecules are left outside (only the skinny short people are taken up into the hotel lobby). These thyroid cells then turn the iodine (which is actually in the iodide form, but that doesn't matter!) into thyroid hormone which then gets stored in a storage compartment within the thyroid – called colloid – which is like the fatter people going further into the hotel. The thyroid cells have up to 50 times the concentration of iodine than in the bloodstream (higher concentration of skinny short people in the hotel lobby compared to on the street). Whilst the thyroid cells have the highest amount of revolving doors (called the sodium / iodide symporter), there are also some on some other organs such as salivary glands, breast tissue, the gut and also the placenta. Radioactive iodine is never given to pregnant women, because some of it would be taken up by the placenta and then would pass through to the fetus, and could cause damage to a developing baby's thyroid and possibly other organs too. In non-pregnant people some radioiodine is taken up by salivary glands, the breasts and the gut. However the amount of uptake is far, far less than in the thyroid, as there are so much fewer revolving doors on these other organs.

Now, most thyroid cancers have developed from thyroid cells that possess these special revolving doors, and hence most thyroid cancer cells are also good at taking up iodine from the circulation. Because these revolving doors can't tell the difference between radioactive iodine and non-radioactive iodine (a short skinny person looks the same as a short skinny person that has just swallowed something radioactive), these thyroid cancer cells also take up radioactive iodine. Radioactive iodine gives off radioactive particles (beta particles), and a relatively lesser amount of radioactive waves (gamma waves). The beta particles only travel a few millimeters, and so once they are inside the thyroid cell, these particles cause local damage. Imagine a crane and a wrecking ball – it does very effective damage in the vicinity of the crane, but the buildings a block away are left untouched. These particles usually kill the cells that take it up, and do very little damage, if any, to any other tissues. The radioiodine then leaks out of the damaged cells, is filtered out of the bloodstream by the kidneys and then peed out in the urine. Any radioiodine that is not taken up into cells is also quite quickly peed out in the urine.

In addition to the biological excretion of radioiodine from the body, the radioiodine is decaying naturally, all the time. Its half-life is about 1 week. This means that if you had a bucket full of radioiodine, and left it untouched in the bucket, in a week's time the bucket would still be full, but the radioactivity levels would be half what they were a week ago. In another week's time the radioactivity would be a quarter of what it first was, then a week later 1 eighth as radioactive, and a week later 1 sixteenth what it first was, etc. So when someone swallows some radioiodine, the total body levels of radioactivity are at their maximum immediately, but drop down quickly, as it is both being peed out, and decaying naturally. The more thyroid cells that person has, the more radioiodine is taken up into cells and so more radioiodine hangs around for a while. Therefore if you have an intact thyroid gland you stay radioactive for a few weeks (at decreasing levels), whereas if you don't have a thyroid gland (e.g. after thyroid surgery to remove it) the radioactivity level drops down much quicker.

So, if you have thyroid cancer, and it is thought that it might have spread outside the thyroid, then the usual treatment is to remove as much of the thyroid and the thyroid cancer as can be removed by surgery, and any thyroid cells that remain (that are either normal thyroid cells or thyroid cancer cells) can then be treated with radioiodine. By taking a drink or capsule of radioiodine, this should hopefully be taken up into any remaining thyroid cells, and kill them off. This can be viewed as a beautiful way of delivering something that can kill the cancer cell, delivering it right inside the cancer cell, leaving the rest of the body relatively untouched.

*Once they decided I needed radioiodine, my main reaction was interest. I was curious as to how it worked and what I could or couldn't do. It was a wee bit hard to keep a distance from my dog, but otherwise it was fine. I wasn't nervous. Once you know something has to be done, you just have to get on with it.*

As with most beautiful things, there are some caveats. Not all thyroid cells take up radioiodine. The medullary cells, that make calcitonin rather than thyroid hormone, do not take up iodine, and so don't take up radioiodine. This is why radioiodine is ineffective at treating medullary thyroid cancer. Also for thyroid cells to take up radioiodine, they have to have the iodine revolving door on their cell surface. For the doors to be present the cell has to perform quite a complicated process of manufacture of the door, and its insertion onto the cell membrane. Cancer cells tend to not have all the complicated abilities that healthy cells have. Instead they focus on growing and replicating, rather than doing much else. This especially applies to those cancer cells that have mutated and deteriorated so that they are a far cry from being like a healthy thyroid cell and so these cells sometimes don't take up much radioiodine. This explains why for some people, particularly if they have had thyroid cancer for a long time, radioiodine is no longer effective at killing these cells. Another thing to bear in mind is that if you had for example 100 thyroid cancer cells at the start, and most of them (say 98%) were really good at taking up radioiodine, these cells get killed, leaving only 2% of thyroid cancer cells. Whilst it's good that the total number of thyroid cancer cells has been massively reduced, the remaining thyroid cancer cells that have survived are not very able to take up radioiodine. Therefore if these cells go on to multiply and become a problem, then this problem won't be so effectively treated with radioiodine. Thankfully thyroid cancer cells are often slow-growing and as long as most of them are wiped out, having some left is often not a problem, particularly if they just hang around in lymph nodes doing nothing very much. There is also the possibility of further surgery to deal with any clumps of thyroid cancer cells that are not responding to radioiodine and become big enough to require removal.

So, if you have had thyroid cancer, and it has likely been completely removed with your initial surgery, then there is no need for radioiodine. If however, there is likely to be some thyroid cancer cells remaining, then the decision to be taken is whether you might benefit from radioiodine. Importantly this potential benefit needs to be weighed against the potential harm from radioiodine. If benefit is clearly more likely than harm, then the decision is usually straightforward. If it's not clear where the balance lies, then the decision is a bit more tricky.

**Potential benefits of radioiodine**

1) Follow-up of thyroid cancer treatment, using thyroglobulin blood tests.

Once the initial treatment of thyroid cancer has happened (surgery and possibly radioiodine), the next phase is long-term follow-up. This is done to identify any future recurrence so as to treat it as quickly and effectively as possible. The 3 main ways to look for any recurrence are 1) your doctor assessing any symptoms and feeling for lumps in your neck, 2) imaging – usually an ultrasound scan of the neck, and 3) thyroglobulin blood tests.

Thyroid cells release thyroglobulin in to the bloodstream that can be measured with a blood test. If you have no thyroid cancer cells your thyroglobulin should be undetectable. In contrast if you have a large thyroid gland present, your thyroglobulin blood test should be much higher. Therefore looking at what the thyroglobulin level is over time can give a good indication as to how many thyroid cells there are in the body and whether they are multiplying. If a person has had surgery to remove as much of the thyroid as possible (it's almost impossible to remove

100% of thyroid, even with the most skilled thyroid surgeon; some remnants almost always remain), and then has radioiodine to kill off as many remaining cells as possible, then the thyroglobulin level should be low and it should stay low over time if there are no thyroid cells multiplying. If however the thyroglobulin is detectable and rising it indicates that there are thyroid cells present and that they are multiplying. If a patient is on the appropriate amount of thyroid hormone replacement, then there is no good reason for normal thyroid cells to grow. In this setting a rising thyroglobulin usually means that thyroid cancer cells are growing and hence is an important clue for your doctor to consider further imaging and further treatment such as repeat surgery or radioiodine.

If a person has thyroid surgery but does not have radioiodine, then a remnant of thyroid gland can be expected to remain and so their thyroglobulin may not be very low. Whilst a subsequently rising thyroglobulin can still be a clue for thyroid cancer recurrence, because initial levels are not undetectable, it's harder to know what a measurable thyroglobulin means. It could mean the presence of remaining healthy thyroid cells not fully removed at surgery, or it could mean presence of thyroid cancer cells.

Therefore, having radioiodine after thyroidectomy surgery can help with future follow-up, making it more clear what a measurable or rising thyroglobulin actually means. One important caveat to this is that some people have proteins in their blood called anti-thyroglobulin antibodies. These probably don't do very much, but one thing they can do is interfere with the blood test that measures thyroglobulin. These antibodies can mop up thyroglobulin so the blood test can't measure it, so the thyroglobulin result is falsely low. Therefore if you have high anti-thyroglobulin antibodies in your blood, then you and your doctor can't rely on a low thyroglobulin blood test result.

2) Reduce the chance of thyroid cancer recurrence

If radioiodine kills off a large proportion of thyroid cancer cells, then this often results in a lower rate of thyroid cancer recurrence in future. Quite who does, and who does not benefit in this way, is a trickier question to answer. The studies are varied and complex, and in-depth discussion of this is probably outside the scope of this book. In general the more advanced the thyroid tumor, the more likely the person is to benefit from radioiodine, including reducing the chance of thyroid cancer recurrence. However, thyroid cancer recurrence doesn't have nearly the same consequences that a recurrence of other tumors might have (like breast cancer, bowel cancer, etc.). A recurrence of thyroid cancer can often be thought of as an unwelcome but not entirely unexpected, nor disastrous, pain-in-the-backside.

A useful comparison is a flat tire in a bicycle race. All bike-racers know this can happen, but other than looking after your tires and steering around visible obstacles, there's not a great deal you can do to avoid it. If you spend the whole race worrying about a potential flat tire, you're not likely to perform well, you'll probably get distracted from your wider goals (placing well in the race, getting more race experience, getting more points for the season that will count towards your final position), and almost certainly worrying about getting a flat tire will reduce your enjoyment of the whole experience. When a flat tire does occur, you immediately know it – your grip goes, both you and the tire feel deflated. Very occasionally this flat tire is bad news – if it blows just as you are going fast round a corner and a truck is coming the other way, the outcome is not good for all concerned. However, this is really rare, usually you just slow up, resign yourself to not being able to compete in that particular race, get the tire fixed and then enjoy the cruise to the finish line knowing that the pressure is off, at least for that race. You'll be back next weekend to go again.

Similarly with thyroid cancer recurrence – very rarely it is significantly bad news, and the truck analogy speaks for itself. However, much more commonly a recurrence is just an unwelcome obstacle to overcome. It may mean more close monitoring, more frequent clinic visits, and probably some form of treatment such as repeat surgery and / or repeat radioiodine. Whilst none of this is welcome, for most people this treatment is enough to knock the disease in the guts, and it shrinks away again, and life goes on. It may recur again in 1 year, 5 years, 20 years, but the usual outcome is that it is kept at bay sufficiently well so that you don't have symptoms from it, and it doesn't go on to significantly impact upon the quality or quantity of your living.

Therefore whilst reducing the risk of thyroid cancer recurrence with radioiodine is a good thing, it's not the all or nothing thing that must be aimed for, irrespective of the cost.

3) Reduce the chance of dying from thyroid cancer

Radioiodine, given in the correct setting, can reduce the risk of dying from thyroid cancer. However, if your thyroid cancer has only a tiny chance of cutting your life short, then reducing a tiny chance to an even smaller chance is unlikely to be of any benefit to you. If you have a 1 in a 1000 chance of dying from thyroid cancer, and radioiodine reduces this risk by half (to 1 in 2000), then you only have a 1 in 2000 chance of radioiodine saving your life. Hugely important, but vanishingly unlikely. In contrast, if you have a 1 in 10 chance of dying from your thyroid cancer, and radioiodine reduces this chance by half (to 1 in 20) then you have a 1 in 20 chance of being the person whose life is saved by radioiodine. Hugely important, and much more likely for you to benefit.

This illustrates that radioiodine needs to be given in the correct setting in order for you to have a reasonable chance of it saving your life. In general, the less advanced the thyroid cancer, the less likely it is to threaten your life, and hence the less likely you are to benefit from radioiodine. One caveat is that, as discussed in the previous chapter, the opposite is not always true. By this I mean that the more advanced thyroid cancers, are sometimes less likely to take up radioiodine, and so the benefits may not be as great as hoped for.

## Potential harm of radioiodine

1) Inconvenience of radioiodine

Radioiodine is inconvenient, particularly if you have close contact with young children or pregnant women. If you have taken radioiodine you'll be excreting radioiodine in your bodily fluids, particularly your urine. You'll also be emitting gamma radiation that will be shining out of you like an invisible light. The inconvenience comes from the fact that you will have to limit the amount of radiation that other people receive from you, both from your body fluids and from you shining out gamma rays on them.

The rules and regulation around this vary from country to country, reflecting that no-one knows for sure what best to do. This is not because no-one cares, but more because the amount of radiation involved is relatively so low that it's very difficult to know whether and to what degree any harm can come from this low level of radiation.

Your own hospital should give you detailed guidance on what to do and what not to do, depending partly on the amount of radioiodine given. The lower doses can be given as an outpatient. This involves you coming into hospital, swallowing a drink of radioactive water or radioactive capsule, and then you leave the hospital. For the higher doses you may need to stay in a specially designed hospital room for a few days, until you have peed out enough radioiodine that your radioactivity levels are low enough for you to be out and about.

You'll be asked to avoid close, prolonged contact with others for a number of days. Close contact usually means within 6 feet (2 metres), and prolonged means more than 5-10 minutes. This means brief contact – a quick chat in the supermarket, passing people in the corridor, a hug goodnight, is all fine. It's like sunburn – you can't get sunburnt if you're only in the sun briefly, but if you're exposed to the sun for hours, you're more likely to receive enough sunrays to cause you some harmful effects. You'll need to sleep in a separate bed from others for a few days, and to avoid going to work for a similar period, but the number of days depends on the type of work you do (e.g. kindergarten teacher versus solitary lighthouse keeper). The length of time you need to stay away from children under 10 years, and pregnant women, will be longer than the time needed to stay away from other adults.

You'll also be advised how to best keep your body fluids to yourself, again for a number of days. Since most of your thyroid gland has been removed by this stage, you won't take up much of the radioiodine, and so you'll excrete it relatively quickly. Most of it will end up in your urine, so you need to avoid urinating on other people – this is not usually a problem, but you meet all kinds of people in this line of work! You should pee down the toilet, and men should sit to pee, to limit any off-target or splashing issues. It's probably best to flush the toilet twice to get the radioactivity down the pipes, where it gets diluted and decays naturally and so can't cause harm to others. Simple hygiene measures usually avoids significant contamination on hands. Crockery and cutlery should be washed before others use them, as your saliva will be radioactive, and whilst it's extremely unlike that a tiny drop of your saliva could do anyone else any harm, it's best avoided. Likewise handling food intended for others with your sweaty hands is not a great idea. Nor is sweating all over your favorite exercise bike at the local gym.

Because you will be an emitter of gamma rays, much like a torch is an emitter of light, you won't leave a radiation memory in the place you previously were. So like a torch no longer illuminates a room that it is no longer in, if you leave the lounge and go to the kitchen, there won't be any radiation left in the lounge (unless you accidently urinated in the lounge, and left a puddle of radioactive pee!).

There are lots of questions that usually arise around precautions to take after radioiodine, many of which will be particular to you and your situation. You should discuss all these issues with your own physician who is licensed to give radioiodine – most doctors won't know much about this. Most of this requires a bit of planning, especially if you are usually in close contact with young children. You won't glow in the dark, and you won't grow 3 heads, and you'll feel fine, but the *idea* of swallowing something radioactive is usually much more difficult than actually doing it.

2) Side effects of radioiodine

For the radioiodine to work best you want the maximum amount of radioiodine to be taken up into any remaining thyroid cells. The iodide transporter (the revolving door in the hotel) works better in the presence of a hormone called TSH (thyroid stimulating hormone). This stimulates the thyroid cells to suck up more radioiodine – the revolving door spins faster, and the hotel lobby gets packed. One way to get the body to increase TSH levels is to have low thyroid hormone levels. This is done by stopping thyroid hormone replacement (T4, thyroxine) a month before the date of radioiodine. However this can make people feel tired, cold and sometimes a bit miserable. This can be minimized by taking a shorter-acting thyroid hormone (T3) for the two weeks after stopping thyroxine, and only going without the T3 for the 2 weeks prior to radioiodine. The T3 levels drop more quickly than the T4, and so just prior to radioiodine both T4 and T3 levels are low, and in response the TSH is high, so encouraging radioiodine uptake. This means that most people feel a bit tired at the time of radioiodine – not due to the radioiodine, but due to being short of thyroid hormone at the time of taking the radioiodine. The thyroxine is then restarted after the radioiodine and the person gradually feels better. About 4 to 6 weeks later they typically feel fully back to normal.

The other way to get a high TSH is to have a TSH injection shortly before the radioiodine. This man-made TSH is expensive and not available in all countries, but using it avoids the tiredness around the time of radioiodine that is caused by the thyroid hormone withdrawal.

Once the radioiodine is swallowed, it gets absorbed from the gut and into the bloodstream from where it gets taken up into cells that possess the iodide transporter. This includes the salivary glands, and having a dry mouth is one of the things that can occur after radioiodine, but it's generally uncommon. That said, it's probably more likely with repeated large doses of radioiodine, and can be permanent, which is annoying, and can make subsequent tooth decay more likely.

3) Chance of radioiodine causing future cancer

Radioactivity can cause cancer. The lower the dose of radioactivity, the lower the chance of causing cancer, and likewise the higher the dose of radioactivity the more likely it is to cause cancer. The radioactive particles and rays can cause damage to the recipe book of a cell (its DNA), and if the recipe is wrong the meal doesn't turn out like it should. If the DNA is damaged the cell might be able to repair itself, or it might die, or it might turn cancerous.

At low radiation doses this either causes insufficient damage to do anything, or the cell repairs itself. We get exposed to radiation every day and over time we accumulate gradually increasing DNA damage. If we are exposed to additional radiation then our DNA is prematurely aged, and the chance of cancer gets brought forward in time. Whilst the amount of radioactivity that you might emit to others having taken radioiodine is generally very small, the do's and don'ts mentioned above are aimed at minimizing exposure to others so their DNA is left undamaged. Obviously if a person is given such a big dose of radioiodine that they get sufficient radiation to cause a second cancer, then this defeats the purpose of giving the radioiodine to try to cure the original thyroid cancer. The decision to use radioiodine takes into account the likely benefits from the radioiodine (such as improved follow-up, reduced chance of thyroid cancer recurrence, and reduced chance of death from thyroid cancer) and balances this against the chance of harm (the increased risk of a second cancer caused by the radioiodine).

The chance of radioiodine causing a second cancer is relatively small. To put it into perspective, when someone is born into this world, assuming they have the good fortune to be born into a stable country with reasonably good sanitation, vaccination, healthcare, etc., about 1 third (33%) of those individuals will ultimately die from cancer. The leading causes include breast cancer, lung cancer and bowel cancer. If an individual is given a relatively large amount of radioiodine (6000MBq), then this increases that individual's future chance of dying from a second cancer that has been caused by the radioiodine by about 1%. Therefore that individual's risk of dying from cancer has gone up from 33% to 34%. You would therefore have to treat 100 people with 6000MBq of radioiodine for 1 of them to die from the radioiodine. You would therefore hope that more than 1 person is prevented from dying of their thyroid cancer by the radioiodine, in order for the benefit of the radioiodine to be greater than the harm from the radioiodine. This is why it's important that the group of patients whom are given this amount of radioiodine are at significant risk of dying from their thyroid cancer, and that radioiodine can indeed save a proportion of them.

The evidence from numerous studies has been brought together to make guidelines which help identify those patients most likely to benefit from radioiodine, and these guidelines take into account the size and stage of the tumor, and how spread it is, etc. The American Thyroid Association has published excellent guidelines to help with the decision of whether radioiodine is likely to be of net benefit.

It's worth noting that the typical dose of radioiodine given is around 1100Mbq (given as an out-patient, where the patient takes the radioiodine and can then leave the hospital immediately), or around 3500Mbq (usually given as an in-patient, where the patient stays in hospital for a couple of days to make sure they have peed out a good proportion of the radioiodine before they leave the hospital). Therefore the 1% increased risk of cancer from radioiodine noted above, would only occur after about 5 of the out patient doses or 2 of the inpatient doses. Doses less than the 6000MBq would be expected to have a lower risk of causing cancer, particularly as at the lower end of radioiodine doses the amount of DNA repair is such that there is no measurable increased risk of future cancer.

Having said all of this, the decision about whether or not to have radioiodine is often fairly easy. Many people clearly have such early stage disease that they are likely to be fully cured by their surgery, or their outlook is so good that radioiodine will not be offering any improvement in an already excellent likely outcome. Alternatively, some people plainly have significant disease where there will be clear benefit from the radioiodine, and there is little doubt about the best course of action. If you are in one of these two groups then the radioiodine decision is pretty straightforward, and becomes just one of the many steps mapped out in front of you. Perhaps one you would rather not take, but at least the path is clear, without too many forks in the road.

*I was really disappointed when I found out that I needed radioiodine. I'd had it in my head that I wouldn't need it, so it was difficult when I found out it was needed. If I'd been prepared from the start that radioiodine was likely, then it would have been easier to take.*

There is of course the group in the middle, where the benefit from radioiodine may be less clear-cut. Factors like the ease of follow-up may become more important, and a lower radioiodine dose given as an out-patient may be a good option. Here your thyroid specialist should be able to advise what best to do. A good question to ask of them may be: "if you were in my shoes, what would you do and why?". The best path should become clear. Even if the best path still seems hard to choose, this may well be because either direction is equally good. If the decision is really tough to call, then it probably doesn't matter which option you pick – the outcome will likely be very similar. For example if you have a relatively low stage cancer, and it's unclear whether radioiodine will help, and you choose to have radioiodine, and you have a future thyroid cancer recurrence, then likely options may include further surgery and/or radioiodine. If you didn't have radioiodine, then you would still have that recurrence and future options may include further surgery and/or radioiodine. The outcome will likely be similar. Therefore if the radioiodine decision is difficult, then that's probably because the outcome will be similar either way, and so in the bigger picture there are probably better things for you to be spending your time, emotions and energy on. Once you have all the necessary facts, have had the necessary discussions and advice from your specialist, then the decision usually makes itself, or if it's not clear, make a decision knowing that the outcome is likely to be similar whatever the decision, and move on to the next step.

The next step is either taking the radioiodine – now that you've got this far, this will be like a walk in the park – or not taking radioiodine (in which case skip the next chapter).

*"Don't be afraid to take a big step when one is indicated. You can't cross a chasm in two small steps"*

David Lloyd George

## Chapter 8 - Taking radioiodine.

Now that you've made the decision to take radioiodine, actually taking it is the easy part. There is no desperate time urgency to receive radioiodine. Thyroid cancer is usually very slow growing, and has likely been present for years prior to its detection. Usually it's wise to leave some time to fully recover from your operation, and generally a 2 to 4 month time frame after surgery for getting your radioiodine is reasonable.

*I wasn't scared of the radioiodine. I was so delighted that I didn't need to be admitted to hospital for it, that I was quite happy about it. It was a bit weird having to stay away from the kids, but at least I was able to be at home, and I wasn't allowed to cook for 3 days, which was great!*

There are 2 potential things to prepare yourself for:
1) a sense of anti-climax when it comes to taking it as an outpatient
2) the boredom of taking it as an in-patient (you may need a good book)

The aim of the game is to get any remaining thyroid cancer cells to suck up as much radioiodine as possible. Whether they are healthy thyroid cells or thyroid cancer cells, we want them to suck up the radioiodine so that as many of these cells as possible are wiped out. For this to happen we want the iodide/sodium transporter (the revolving hotel door) to be working overtime, so that it welcomes as much radioiodine as possible into the thyroid cells. This revolving door works faster in the presence of a hormone called TSH.

The 2 ways of getting high TSH levels at the time of taking the radioiodine are:

1) stop taking thyroid hormone for a few weeks

2) get an injection of TSH


Your own hospital will have its own way of getting your TSH up. Option 1 is very effective and much cheaper, but can make you feel quite tired by the time you take the radioiodine because your thyroid hormone levels (the FT4 and FT3) will be low. It also takes a number of weeks for your energy levels to return to normal after you re-start your thyroid hormone replacement. Option 2 is effective, but more expensive, and doesn't make you feel tired like option 1. Both options work well, and it may be the financial situation of you and/or your hospital/healthcare system that determines which is available to you.


Once your TSH is up, and you are ready for your radioiodine, you will likely have some blood tests, and if you are female and of fertile age you will need a pregnancy test to make sure you are not pregnant (if you are pregnant, the radioiodine will be postponed until after pregnancy). The level of thyroglobulin immediately prior to taking the radioiodine can be a helpful guide as to what total volume of thyroid cells you may have in your body just prior to the radioiodine. This level can be compared to later thyroglobulin levels to get a rough guide of what proportion of thyroid cells were wiped out by the radioiodine (this is assuming you don't have high levels of anti-thyroglobulin antibodies, which can mess with the thyroglobulin blood test result).

## Out-patient radioiodine

If you are having the radioiodine as an out-patient, you'll then get a drink or capsule of radioiodine. Both do the same thing. The drink tastes of whatever your hospital dilutes the few drops of radioiodine into. We use water, so our radioiodine drink tastes of water. There's no good reason why yours couldn't be a gin and tonic. The capsule is usually quite small and has a smooth coating, and is easily swallowed (don't chew it!), and washed down with water (or gin and tonic). At this point you may feel a sense of anti-climax, because that is it. No pain, no dramas, nothing, and you just walk straight out of the hospital. You will have been given advice about what to do and not to do in the days following the radioiodine. The details of this vary slightly from country to country, and more importantly they vary depending on your home situation, job, etc. They will likely involve you avoiding close contact (within 6 feet) with others for a period of time, and will probably advise you taking particular care to avoid close contact with young children and pregnant women in order to minimize any radiation exposure to others.

You will also be advised how to keep your bodily fluids to yourself, particularly your urine, as you will be excreting most of the radioiodine out down the toilet. Those in the habit of peeing anywhere else than down the toilet will need to curtail these habits, at least for a while! Because there is not likely to be large amounts of thyroid tissue in your body following your thyroidectomy, most of the radioiodine doesn't get taken up into cells and gets peed straight out, hence your radiation levels drop very quickly, and the length of time you need to avoid close contact with others and be careful with your bodily fluids is usually days rather than weeks.

**In-patient radioiodine**

If you are having an in-patient dose of radioiodine, this is usually because the radioiodine dose chosen is a bit higher, and there are various rules that dictate what dose can be given as an in-patient or out-patient. Being an inpatient for radioiodine can be boring, although some find it relaxing. You will likely be admitted to a special radiation-protected room, so that the gamma rays that you are shining out do not get through the walls of your room and so they don't shine on the other patients in the adjacent rooms. Your bodily fluids will need to go down your designated toilet, and your bedclothes and other items that you may have sweat on, or urinated on, or otherwise contaminated will have to be treated in a special way (this usually involves storing them in a radiation-containing room somewhere for 1 month, after which the radiation levels will have naturally decayed to about 1/16$^{th}$ of the original level due to the half-life of radioiodine[131] being about 1 week).

During your inpatient stay you won't have direct contact with others. Meals may well be delivered through a hatch, and you won't be allowed visitors although most facilities have telephones or wi-fi access to allow at least electronic contact with others. You may well be quite bored, and if you have been off thyroid hormone for a few weeks you may also be quite tired. This time can be quite relaxing – you are forced to take time out from the day-to-day stresses of life. It can be a time to read that book you have not got round to reading. Because it is forced isolation time, it may well be worth giving some thought as to how to get the most out of it. For some 2 days of forced rest is just what they need!

*The radioiodine was quite a hard time – I had to be isolated from my children. My children and my husband moved in with my parents and I stayed at home on my own. I felt a bit lonely, but my brother and husband came to visit – we talked, but from a distance. I read a lot. I did a lot of thinking. I looked back a lot at all the time I had spent in this world. I actually found it the best time to do some thinking, to give me a rest spiritually, and during that time I decided to live my life a bit differently from then on. I wanted to live a peaceful, a pure life, full of love, and contributing to my society, to the whole universe.*

You'll likely be in hospital for 2 or 3 days. At the end of your stay the physicist in the hospital may take some measurements to make sure your radiation levels have dropped down to the expected level prior to you being discharged. Then you head home.

Whether you have radioiodine as an in-patient or an outpatient, the potential adverse effects are similar. Generally they are very few. Some people can get a dry mouth, particularly if they have had repeated doses because it can get taken up into the salivary glands and cause a reduction in the amount of saliva that can then be produced. I always found it surprising that there is rarely any pain involved. Presumably because the thyroid cell deposits don't have a good nerve supply (if any). Even in hyperthyroid patients who have their whole thyroid intact, who are getting radioiodine to try to zap the whole gland, even this group of patients rarely gets any thyroid pain. The occasional patient experiences some nausea with radioiodine, but I'm reluctant even to mention this because I'm guessing that many of these people experience nausea as part of the nervous reaction to the idea of taking radioiodine, rather than a physical response to the actual radioiodine. Vomiting up the radioiodine is not ideal as it means only a proportion gets in to the body to do its thing, and the rest needs to be cleaned up by the men in white coats.

We once had a patient who had an out-patient dose of radioiodine, who then was travelling home as a passenger in a car. After about 1 hour she got nauseous (probably travel sickness). They pulled over and she vomited at the side of the road, by a field, not sure exactly where, and then they drove on. When she got home she phoned us to tell about it. We had to send the men in the white coats out in a car with a Geiger counter, trying to identify the particular field where she had deposited her radioactive vomit. After some searching they found the mound, and had to dig it up, and retrieve it in a lead container and bring it back to the hospital to be stored for a month for it to decay into very smelly, but no longer radioactive, vomit. It is not wise to leave radioactive vomit out in the community, in case wildlife, or pets eat it, or children stumble across it, or by some other means people get unintentionally exposed to radiation.

The lessons from this episode are not to expect nausea from radioiodine, to avoid anything that might make you nauseous (rollercoaster rides, etc.), and that if vomiting is unavoidable, even with the help of anti-nausea medication, then try to vomit down a toilet!

No matter whether you had in-patient or out-patient radioiodine, this treatment is usually followed by an iodine uptake scan a few days later, often referred to as a post-ablative scan. This involves you lying under a big camera that detects gamma rays. If radioiodine has been taken up into any thyroid cells, it will stay in those cells for a number of days while it is zapping the cells from the inside with the beta particles that the radioiodine gives off. These particles only travel a short distance (a few mm) and so effectively zap the thyroid cells and leave the rest of you relatively untouched. The radioiodine also gives out a smaller amount of gamma rays, and these zip out of the body and can be detected by a gamma camera. Therefore if you have a big enough collection of thyroid cells (for example a lymph node containing thyroid cancer cells) these can give off enough gamma rays for the node to be detected by the gamma camera, and so show up on the post-ablative scan. Whilst this scan is not a high-definition scan (it's usually just a collection of fuzzy grey dots), it can give some useful information as to whether and where the radioiodine was taken up. If some areas show up on the scan then this may indicate where thyroid cells are located, and hopefully these areas will have been zapped by the radioiodine that was taken up there. If there is no uptake visible on the scan then either the volume of cancer cells is so little that they weren't visible, or that the thyroid cells there are not taking up radioiodine. The scan can sometimes be difficult to interpret as radioiodine can appear in certain areas (like the bowel, salivary glands, etc.) and so sometimes it can be difficult to tell whether the dots on the scan are due to thyroid cells or normal cells. Having said all that, this scan is often useful, and the information gathered is added to all your other information to gain a better picture of where things are at, and what the best next steps are.

Now, it's all eyes forward to the next stage, which is life with thyroid cancer, and how to make it better.

"If you're reading this...
Congratulations, you're alive.
If that's not something to smile about,
then I don't know what is."


Chad Sugg, a poem from Monsters Under Your Head

# Chapter 9 - Follow-up; life with thyroid cancer and how to start making it better

By now you've come a long way.

You've had your initial symptoms, gone to see someone about them, had the initial assessment, and the necessary tests. You've had your FNA, and had to deal with the diagnosis and all the fear and uncertainty that comes with that. Then there was probably more scans, then surgery and then you had to deal with the details of how widespread the thyroid cancer may be. Then there was possible radioiodine, and additional scans. Surely you must be through the worst by now?

The answer is typically mixed; yes and no.

Yes, the majority of initial stages are behind you. You've probably had a number of months to try to get your head around things, punctuated by the various tests and procedures which may focus you on the present, prevent you from denying the whole thing, but may also distract you from the bigger picture, the longer game. Now that the initial rollercoaster is behind you, the challenge is to face the future. This can be both a challenge and an opportunity, and is perhaps your greatest chance to make some positive and pro-active changes that will help you to live a better life from here on, each and every day, no matter what the outcome from your thyroid cancer. Although this might sound contradictory or counter-intuitive, it's one of the real positives that can come out of your illness. This is discussed more in Chapter 11, but for now we'll cover some of the follow-up issues.

## Follow-up

The practicalities of follow-up for your thyroid cancer are fairly straightforward, and involve a 3-pronged approach to look for any signs of tumor recurrence or tumor progression. The 3 prongs are 1) your thyroid specialist feeling in your neck for any lumps and bumps that shouldn't be there, 2) having a thyroglobulin blood test, 3) having a scan of your neck, usually an ultrasound scan. This will happen at various intervals from a few months to a few years, depending on how your thyroid cancer is behaving.

During this time there might be lots of things to come to terms with. Sometimes even apparently small things might stir up an emotional response – even the name of the clinic might be a trigger.

*The word cancer is part of the problem. Everyone in society thinks cancer means the same thing. Even though I know that it's not all the same, the word is still very emotive. Even my appointment letter has Thyroid Cancer Clinic written on it, and even after all I've been through and all that I now know about thyroid cancer, that word still gets to me. Each time the letter arrives I show it to my husband and say – look at it! You can't forget that, can you! I wish they'd call it something else!*

Generally the intervals between appointments stretch out if the cancer is behaving in a very slow-growing way or if it's thought to be likely cured. Even in those patients where it's thought likely that there are very few if any thyroid cells remaining, there is the odd person in whom the thyroid cancer shows up many years down the track, which is why follow-up is generally lifelong.

It's worth bearing in mind that thyroid cancer usually behaves very differently from many other cancers. If thyroid cancer does return many years after being thought to have been cured, this is more like an unwelcome obstacle to be overcome, rather than a major disaster. Even in this late recurrence situation, the disease is usually controllable, with the help of radioiodine and surgery, and the chance of it having a significant effect on your quality or quantity of life remains surprisingly low. It is sometimes quite difficult to get your head around this, as it is so different to what may be the case with many other cancers. With some other cancers a future recurrence of the disease can signify a return of disease that is often extremely difficult to control and such a return of those cancers often heralds the last stages of the person's life. Understanding this difference between most thyroid cancers, and these other types of cancer is an important positive for thyroid cancer patients to get their head around, but also for their friends and family.

These 3 monitoring prongs of 1) feeling, 2) blood test & 3) scanning, are in addition to you seeing and talking with your thyroid specialist who should be not only checking for symptoms of thyroid cancer, but also listening to you and helping you deal with any other issues that might be affecting your health. In many healthcare systems, time is short, and appointments with specialists are short, and there may not be sufficient time or headspace for all the issues to be dealt with. It is often easier, and the only practical way for your specialist to cope with their workload, if they have a fairly blinkered and focused approach, skipping quickly to the 3 prongs of monitoring. If things are going well with your thyroid cancer then this is often an acceptable situation – fairly short, sharp, business-like appointments, every 6 to 12 months, offering reassurance that everything's OK. This deals with the necessary medical issues, but may miss the importance of emotional and other issues. In this situation it may be that your GP/family physician can offer additional support.

There may be others around you that can help, such as friends and family, and other health professionals such as cancer nurse specialists, clinical psychologists and trained counselors. If things are not going so well with your thyroid cancer then your specialist should make the time to listen and answer your questions as best they can. This is often when it helps to have a friend or family member present with you in the appointment to help remember what is being said, and to help ask the questions that need to be answered. Having a list of important questions written before the appointment is often a useful way to make sure that you get what you need out of the consultation.

**Living with cancer in your neck**

Thyroid cancer is weird, in a relatively good way, in that it usually grows very slowly. The aim of treatment is to prevent the disease from having anything more than the minimum possible negative impact on your quality and quantity of life. The initial treatment (the surgery and possibly radioiodine) aims to get rid of as many thyroid cancer cells as possible, and the on-going follow-up aims to keep whatever is left from negatively affecting your life. When thyroid cancer does return, it is often because there was a small cluster of cancer cells hiding somewhere (usually in lymph nodes in the neck), and these have grown to noticeable size over the following months and years. The usual gut reaction to the news that there is a cluster of cancer cells in your neck is to want to have them removed/killed/wiped out as soon as possible. Of course this is the natural response! – get them out now! This is based on our general understanding that cancer is bad, and it needs to be removed before it spreads anywhere else. This is usually true because many cancers grow fast and cause disruption and trouble wherever they are growing, the more they grow the more they spread, and the more trouble they cause. But thyroid cancer is different. It usually grows very slowly.

The concept of a slowly growing cancer is challenging, but the understanding of that concept needs to be brought into decision-making regarding thyroid cancer treatment, and in particular the timing of treatment.

In a nutshell the main treatment of thyroid cancer recurrence is either surgery or radioiodine, or both. As a general rule of thumb if there are lymph nodes in the neck containing cancer, and these nodes are more than a centimeter in short axis diameter*, then surgery to pluck these out is often the best approach. On the other hand if there is evidence of lots of small tumor deposits, and particularly if they are in places difficult to get at with surgery, then radioiodine is often the best approach. A combination of both approaches is often used – i.e. surgery to pluck out what can be plucked out from the neck, and the radioiodine to try to wipe out as much as possible of what cells are left – similar to the initial treatment of your thyroid cancer. These treatments usually significantly reduce the total number of thyroid cancer cells, and it may be years or even decades before what remains grows enough to need to do anything about it.

*this centimeter is in front to back diameter, not head to foot diameter because long, thin upright lymph nodes lying in a head to foot direction are often benign*

There are only so many times that surgery to the neck is a good idea. With each surgery it becomes technically more difficult, with increasing scar tissue from the previous surgeries, and the anatomy becoming a bit distorted. With each additional operation, the chance of causing harm from the operation increases – such as bleeding, infection, injury to the nerve to the voice, injury to the parathyroid glands causing low blood calcium levels. Plus there is the repeated exposure to general anesthetics which are best avoided if possible.

There is also a limit on how often you can have radioiodine, as the greater the total dose of radioiodine, the greater the chance of causing a cancer in the future. As mentioned previously, you have to be fairly sure that you are much more likely to experience benefit from radioiodine (killing off thyroid cancer cells), than you are to suffer harm from radioiodine (causing a different cancer).

Therefore the 2 main weapons for keeping thyroid cancer under control (surgery and radioiodine) need to be unleashed at the right time – not too early, not too late, and not to frequently. Given that our foe, the thyroid cancer, is often growing very slowly and causing no trouble, it makes no sense to repeatedly operate to pluck out a tiny lump of fairly inert cells, or to have repeated radioiodine to try to reduce the number of thyroid cancer cells if those cells are not doing very much.

The best strategy for a low-volume recurrence of thyroid cancer may well be to just watch and wait. To wait until is it big enough to be worth doing something about. This watching and waiting can be a head-wrecker, if it's not viewed in the right way – i.e. as the best tactic at the time in the long game of keeping the thyroid cancer under control, and deploying our limited-use weapons at the best possible moment.

## The emotional burden of thyroid cancer

Whilst it's impossible for this short book to cover all the possible follow-up scenarios for you and your cancer, one big part of disease follow-up that is often largely overlooked by the medical profession is the emotional burden of the whole thing. I don't mean to overly criticize the medical profession – I'm sure that the vast majority of healthcare workers are doing their very best to be understanding, and empathetic, but I don't think most medical professionals are really in a position to properly understand how it feels to be you, in your situation. It's likely that most of them (myself included) think they are doing a pretty good, holistic job, especially given the time constraints – they may only have 10 or 15 minutes to cover all that needs to be covered. It was only after I was faced with being in a comparable situation – i.e. having a totally unexpected potentially life-threatening condition, and having to go through the medical maze of tests, and waits, and anxiety and fear and consultations, that I got even an inkling of how far short I had been of understanding what it feels like to be in that situation.

I had not understood that with every test, or scan, or appointment letter, the lid on the deep box of anxiety, fear and emotion gets re-opened. It was probably easier for me than most, given that my diagnosis was made in the hospital that I work in, and I was familiar with the system and many of the people within it. However, one downside was that I could easily access my own medical information. My illness is a type of congenital heart disease, affecting a heart valve and other important structures in that area, which is diagnosed by a heart scan. Having had my first heart scan and unaware of the seriousness of the problem, I looked up my own heart scan result. I can vividly remember clicking on the icon on the computer screen, and up popped the first and most serious diagnosis I had ever faced, with a likely outcome of my life being shortened, but uncertainly so (I could live anywhere from 1 year to 30 years). In that moment I had to face the fact that I was not going to live forever, and indeed I might not live to see my children grow up, or even get to high school. To this day I cannot click on the icon of a patient's heart scan, without having that same emotional response – fear, sweaty, heart racing, etc. It gets less intense with time but it remains real and palpable and unpleasant, even though this is looking up other patient's scans as part of my everyday work. I now never look up my own scans, which occur every 6 months.

Getting some understanding of this helped me realize, that at least for some people, the whole emotional burden of thyroid cancer follow-up, can be huge. Wherever possible we now try to minimize delays between scans or blood tests and follow-up appointments, or try to phone patients when appropriate, to try to reduce the amount of time people have to wait in uncertainty, wondering where things are at. We try to at least acknowledge that follow-up can be difficult, even when it is going well. It forces things back up to the surface, which have been fairly happily buried away since the last appointment.

*I used to get scans every year, but now it's every 2 years, so thank goodness I get more of a break. When you come up for review, it's absolutely all you think about. I'm a very compartmentalized thinker and between clinics I can lock it away. But when the clinic letter arrives, it all starts again.*

This brings us on to how a person deals with the uncertainty and the life-long issue of having had, or actually still having, thyroid cancer. Earlier I referred to the box of negative emotions that go along with my own condition, whose lid gets opened prior to each scan or appointment. Also for some the concept of having things 'buried' as a coping strategy is often used. Both of these techniques involve containing emotions and thoughts; keeping them deep enough down, or tightly enough locked away, that they don't obviously affect our day-to-day lives. Such techniques are often useful, particularly in the short term, when the priority is just to survive the now. However, for many, keeping things buried or locked away is not the best way to go if longer-term inner peace and happiness is the aim. These things are rarely buried deeply enough that they never surface from time to time, even in the subconscious. They are rarely locked away securely enough that no part of it can escape from time to time.

*Most of the time my thyroid cancer worries are fully locked away, especially at work, but at home, with my family, it's never fully buried. My husband likes to keep normality, which is perhaps a bit of denial behavior. But there are times when things are a bit shit for me, and I need to be given a bit of a break. Don't expect too much of me because actually I have had this, and I have had that, and it's not easy.*

*I don't think about future thyroid cancer treatment until I receive my thyroid clinic appointment letter. That's a month before the appointment. So I end up worrying for one month out of twelve – that's a twelfth of my life.*

An alternative approach is to try to reach a state of genuine acceptance, a state of inner peace, where there is no need to keep things buried or hidden away – you are fully accepting of them, and so they hold no power over you, and are free to fly away. But how an individual gets to that point is another question. For me, I had to accept the prospect of risky open-heart surgery, and the possibility of premature heart failure, stroke and death. – Easy!

*I think everything happens for a reason, and now I just accept it. It's taken me at least 6 months from diagnosis to get to that point. At first I felt angry and upset, and even a bit ashamed. I'm not sure why. I didn't want other people to know, I didn't want them feeling sad for me, or my news upsetting them.*

The prospect that I might face major, potentially life-limiting health problems before my children reached high school, is so far from what I had imagined my future would hold that it seemed highly unlikely that I would ever be truly accepting of it. This brings us to the idea that one's happiness is related to the difference between our expectations and our reality. If I am expecting a long, healthy life, with a satisfying career, loving family, and early retirement full of doting grandchildren and foreign travel, then that is such a big ask (and also such a statistically unlikely outcome compared to the history of outcomes for human existence) that it's quite likely that my reality will fall short of that, and so I will not be happy. On the other hand if I am expecting a short, miserable existence with a fair amount of suffering on the way, then I am more likely to be happy with my lot, because there's more chance that my life will fulfill or even surpass my expectations. So one of the aspects which gives weight to the buried or locked up emotions, is the long term expectations, even if they have never been actually fully defined or verbalized. If your expectations can be brought more to the present rather than the future, then this sometimes makes the difference between reality and previous expectation less of a gulf. For example if the hope for the day is to wake up (always a good start), and be able to do some of the things you enjoy (e.g. have your favorite thing for breakfast, listen to the radio, see your daughter for lunch, do your best not to be rude to the person who bugs you most at work, and come home to watch your favorite TV program after dinner) – then that may well be an achievable plan for the day.

If you are able to be bring your focus more to the present, to be more mindful of each moment in each day, and of the richness of experience that is there in each moment, then life can be much more enjoyable.

You don't have to have a life-changing diagnosis in order to shift your focus more to the present and the important things in life, but the reality for most of us (myself included) is that in today's modern living it needs something big like thyroid cancer, or some other life-event, to jolt us into action.

*At the start I had decided I would seize the moment, make every day count, but with time I've found I tend to get sucked back in to the rat race! Perhaps that's partly because my thyroid cancer treatment has gone so well that I've never really genuinely been scared that it might limit my life. If I was really fearful about the future then I think I would have made more major changes.*

There are some who didn't need something so unpleasant to motivate positive change (like some Buddhists), and good on them for doing so, but now that something big has happened, what better opportunity to make the most out of today and all future todays?

*'Tragedy should be utilized as a source of strength. No matter what sort of difficulties, how painful experience is, if we lose our hope, that's our real disaster."*

Dalai Lama XIV

# Chapter 10 - When things aren't going so well

## Getting to acceptance

Your experience of thyroid cancer may well be one of ups and downs. Perhaps two steps forwards, then one step back. There will probably be moments of relief, even joy, perhaps when a suspected recurrence is a false alarm, or when a test result is reassuring, and thyroid cancer can be allowed to fade away from immediate consciousness, at least for a while. However, there will almost certainly be moments that are much harder to take. When the news you get is not what you wanted to hear. When the news makes if clearer how wide the gap is between what you were hoping for, and what your likely reality is going to be.

Many of the setbacks you experience will be just that – a setback. Something disappointing that knocks you back, but something that with some re-adjustment can be over-come. Perhaps a recurrence requiring surgery, perhaps another radioiodine treatment. Neither of these things are particularly welcome, but if they are seen as just part of the necessary steps to keep your disease under control so that you can continue to do the things you want to do for as long as you want to do them, then they can be easier to take. With some big-picture thinking it's often possible to get to a point of welcoming the treatment required to deal with each set-back – but that might take lots of practice and support.

However, for most of us, at some point in our lives we will receive news that is more than just a temporary setback. This is true irrespective of whether you have thyroid cancer or not – the exception being those people who pass away from a sudden event of which they had no warning. I have often wondered whether it would be better to succumb to a car crash, or sudden heart attack, with no warning, no time to prepare, or whether it is better to have some degree of advanced warning that days are coming to an end. It's probably too big a question for most of us, and one that we are not generally ever really required to answer. There are benefits of both, although from my own personal and professional experience, in most cases I'd choose some warning. Living with the knowledge that time is precious can help the person get the most out of life, presuming that the person's quality of life is reasonably good. However, a key aspect of this is having real acceptance of one's own situation. Once a person manages to get to the point of acceptance, then life can be far richer and more rewarding than it might otherwise be, even if time is very limited. Getting to the point of acceptance can be really hard, especially for those not aware that this is where they need to get. This is where the stages of grief reaction can be hugely important, because knowledge of these processes and stages, and the awareness that you are going through them and are able to get out the other side, can make the journey so much more comforting and easier for everyone involved.

**Grief reactions**

There is a huge amount written about grief reactions, and different people respond in different ways, with varying amounts of resilience. To cut a long story short, you may well experience some of these well-recognized stages, and knowing a bit about it can help you get successfully through it, to the point of acceptance. Perhaps the most famous description is The Kübler-Ross model, commonly known as the five stages of grief introduced by Elisabeth Kübler-Ross in 1969.

The five stages she described are:

1. Denial
2. Anger
3. Bargaining
4. Depression
5. Acceptance

My favorite explanations of these emotional stages comes from Wikipedia and if you're at all interested I'd suggest you take the time to go on-line and give it a quick read.

(http://en.wikipedia.org/wiki/Kübler-Ross_model)

Importantly, people don't necessarily go through these stages in any particular order, but instead can bob backwards and forwards between the different stages and experiences. A person might even flit in and out of the stages for minutes at a time, or it can take months to truly emerge through a stage. It's as if a person needs a certain amount of time in each stage in order for the issues to be genuinely resolved, in order to allow the person to get to the point of acceptance.

*Up until that clinic appointment no one had asked about the emotional side of it. People had been nice, but they'd never asked about how I felt. I don't think doctors are taught the emotional side, they are taught the cognitive science stuff. I remember up until that time I hadn't realized I was angry. 5 years before I had been* *diagnosed with a brain tumor. But I know that s\*\*t happens, and for me I was really lucky because my tumor was one of the 1% of that type that were not cancerous. So I felt that's OK, I've recovered, but why have I got something else? I'm not even 50 and now I've had two things; that's not fair.*

*So I think I got the anger part of my grief process with the thyroid cancer but hadn't really realized it until I was asked how I actually felt. And I was really angry then. But it helped to talk about it and to acknowledge it, and it kind of makes you recognize your human-ness. You're allowed to feel angry, you're allowed to feel like that, you're allowed to be really pissed off. This doesn't happen to most people, so it's OK to feel like this.*

If you find yourself stuck in one stage of your grief process, and not making any progress, then this can be a useful indicator that the grief process has become maladaptive – so instead of helping the person deal with the life situation, it hinders them. At this point things may have strayed from a 'normal' grief reaction, into clinical depression that may need additional help to treat (such as appropriate counseling and/or medication).

*I was angry, pissed off, sad. But I didn't want to show any of my feelings to my family. I had young children at the time and I didn't want to upset them or worry them. I never cried. I was really upset inside, but I didn't want to use crying to show my feelings. I did talk to my close family, but I mainly told them what treatment I was going to get, rather than the emotional things I was going through.*

Whilst most grief reactions are traditionally linked to the loss of a loved one, a very similar reaction can occur after receiving difficult news regarding one's own future. Receiving difficult news about your own health, be that from thyroid cancer or any other illness, is very much a situation of loss. Your previous hopes and ideas of what your future would hold and the things you would do and see, may well no longer be a reality. The difference between what you had hoped for and what is likely to occur, is a loss, possibly a huge loss, more than enough to trigger a grief reaction. This type of loss is of course less concrete than the loss of a loved one. It is only a potential loss – the difference between your hopes and your reality. Your hopes may have been wildly unrealistic – you were maybe always going to have a fatal heart attack aged 60, and so having thyroid cancer diagnosed at 55 may not shorten your life at all. But if at 55 you were expecting to live to 88 years of age, and to be enjoying parachute jumping until aged 87, then getting thyroid cancer could quite rightly strike you as a huge loss. We usually have no idea what our fate would have been in the absence of thyroid cancer – we probably hadn't given it really serious thought, but never-the-less, being diagnosed with thyroid cancer, or receiving the news that your thyroid cancer is no longer responding to treatment, is solid grounds for experiencing a grief reaction.

*Right at the beginning there's a bit of the 'why-me?'. I don't remember feeling angry, and I wasn't really denying it. I just compartmentalized it and put it to one side. Then later I felt gratitude that things can be done, and then after it all, I just felt blessed that it all went so well.*

The recognition of your own reaction, and your progress through it can really help you and those who care about you understand why you are feeling as you do, and the knowledge that getting to acceptance does make life much easier to deal with can be a crucial aspect of you living better with thyroid cancer.

*"For after all, the best thing one can do when it is raining is let it rain."*

Henry Wadsworth Longfellow

# Chapter 11 - Living better with thyroid cancer

As you will have realized by now, this book is not intended to be a textbook of thyroid cancer. There are plenty of detailed textbooks out there, and lots of (sometimes really good) information on the internet if you want to plough through the details of thyroid cancer. Given the complexity of the subject and the huge range of individual circumstances, this wealth of knowledge is incredibly difficult to navigate through. It usually needs a good healthcare professional who knows the subject and knows your individual situation really well, to help advise what best to do. No textbook can offer the sort of tailored guidance that you need.

*I had tried Googling it. I went on to one site, that lead me on to another site, and another, and they turned out to be contradictory or the cases were really severe, ending in death. You've no idea of the quality of the stuff that's online. Some of the more personal sites rung true, whereas the professional ones I found pretty unhelpful – I didn't know what information applied to me. But you can relate to peoples' feelings.*

However, I have found that whilst many clinicians can offer really good advice, they usually only have the time and skills to deal with the medical aspects, and are less able to deal with all the other issues that come hand-in-hand with having a diagnosis of cancer (or any other potentially life-threatening diagnosis). Whilst it is often said that thyroid cancer is one of the less bad cancers to get, it is often still a huge issue. Just because most thyroid cancer patients do well, doesn't help you if you are not one of that majority. Even if your disease is likely to be well-controlled or even cured, it doesn't mean that the emotional and psychological burden evaporates away. This book is intended to help with your process of dealing with all the other stuff that goes along with having a diagnosis of thyroid cancer.

My own experience as a doctor who treats patients with thyroid cancer, plus also having my own diagnosis has completely changed my perspective. I thought I was reasonably understanding, compassionate and empathetic. It was only after having my own diagnosis that I realized how incomplete and superficial my understanding was of the psychological and emotional impact of being on the receiving end of such a diagnosis. I was probably already at the more empathetic end of the spectrum of doctors before my diagnosis, and even then, looking back I am embarrassed at my well-meaning but naïve approach. The harsh reality is that doctors often don't have enough time to manage the medical issues as well as they would like, let alone have the time (or skills) to address the other stuff. Even if there was time, I don't think I would have been able to be very helpful as without truly experiencing being on the receiving end of bad news regarding your own health, it's hard to imagine ever being able to fully appreciate what that is like.

Having been on the receiving end I now have a better understanding of what helped, and continues to help, me to get through. There are some people who really don't need much help. They seem to be blessed with various characteristics that result in them apparently coping well. Those people probably won't have read this far into this book – they'd be off enjoying themselves! Some people have such strong innate resilience that nothing seems to make them wobble. They can keep a positive perspective and rock on regardless. There are others that deal with things more by denial that is so effective that it genuinely seems to work, at least temporarily. This is probably not such a healthy mechanism, but it can be really effective for getting through a crisis. Then there are the rest of us – a mixture of ordinary people who when faced with a potentially huge life event find things difficult. I think this is normal! Whilst we may have lots of life experience to help us deal with whatever is ahead, most of us that get told we have thyroid cancer will be facing this type of challenge for the first time and in that setting I think it is normal for this to be difficult.

**What helps**

There are a number of things that will help you deal with the psychological challenge of thyroid cancer, and get you to a point where you can actually live better with thyroid cancer, than you did beforehand. Sounds odd, but it is true, at least for some people. Facing thyroid cancer is not just about thyroid cancer, but it's about facing our own mortality. Even though deep down we know death and taxes are the only 2 true unavoidables in life, we likely spend little time really thinking about them, and even if we do we probably think more about our taxes. Whilst we have more and more birthdays, and the number goes up, and those around us grow up, most of us tend to bury our own mortality deep down, and choose to think about other things – often the day-to-day goings-on that are a good distraction from the bigger issues. As with other anxieties, we are often better at identifying the issue, rather than getting beyond it. We see the obstacle, but not the solution. A really good way of minimizing the impact of the obstacle is to go the next step and play out what the options may be. When you put the options into perspective they often don't seem so bad. You then also work out practical ways to make the outcomes of those options better. The end result being that the obstacle itself is not so scary.

As a child I used to get upset at the thought of my dog dying. I was very fond of the dog, it was our first family pet, and we spent many happy hours together. The thought of her dying was so painful that whenever I considered it I felt sick, and scared. It caused me great upset, and certainly limited the enjoyment I was able to experience at the time, because I was scared that the time would end. I wish I had talked to someone about it at the time. They might have been able to help be identify the obstacle (the death of the dog), and then talk me through the options. These might include me being comforted by the fact that when the dog was old, the veterinary care would be excellent, so there would be minimal suffering. It would be painful for me at the time, but things would get better, I might soon be ready to get a new dog, or perhaps focus more on those things that I hadn't been able to do because of the responsibilities of being a dog-owner. That time would heal, and things would be OK. That nothing stays the same, things move on, but things would be OK, different, possibly better, but OK.

Had I been able to talk through those things at the time, then I suspect I would have had been much happier. I wouldn't have felt so sick or scared. I'd have been much more able to enjoy each moment, without the hindrance of my concerns that things might come to an end.

As it happened, the dog lived to a ripe old age, and I had left home and was at University when she finally died. In retrospect it was me who left the dog, rather than the dog leaving me. I think of all the unnecessary negative emotion I had spent on my relationship with my dog – what a waste – we should have just been enjoying our time together while it lasted!

Whilst this story is just that – a true story of a child's relationship with his dog – and is very simplistic and unsophisticated, it does touch on some of the issues that can help us deal with bigger things, including one's own mortality. Deep down we all know that our days are limited. If we manage to truly ignore this, then the preciousness of life cannot be fully appreciated (if diamonds were in unlimited supply, they would no longer be precious). On the other hand if we spend too much time thinking about it in a negative way (i.e. the child being sick and scared at the thought of the dog dying), then that will take away from the pleasures of being alive. The key is to get to a point of balance and peace, such that we are accepting and comfortable with our own mortality, so that the thought of it doesn't make us sick or scared, but where we also are able to allow the appreciation of our impermanence that each day, and all the moments within each day, can be enjoyed and treasured. This can allow us to get so much more out of what time we have, that life can be much better than it was before. It may be that thyroid cancer is the catalyst that forces us to get to this point of balance, and so what in isolation feels like a negative, can actually be used as a force for positivity.

*I'm a live-for-today person, I'm very spontaneous – was I always like that or has it got more since the diagnosis? I think yes, it certainly has got more. Having thyroid cancer has brought it home that life is unpredictable. I now grasp the opportunities and don't worry about money. I'm now embedded in the idea that life is short, life is unpredictable. Perhaps some of that comes from having gone through the medical things I have gone through. It just becomes more clear, the fragility of what's going on.*

I would much rather that someone had sat down with me as a child and helped me to see all this, and supported me to be at peace with my own mortality, and get positivity out of every possible moment. However, you and I can both guess the chances of that actually happening! Even if there had been someone there to talk to me, I doubt that I would have listened or properly understood.

Perhaps for most of us it does have to be a big, negative, life event in order for us to really be shaken up enough to deal with the big stuff. I don't think winning the lottery would have done it – an apparently positive event, but probably with long-term negative consequences. Having thyroid cancer, or congenital heart disease, or whatever, is the mirror image of this – i.e. an apparently negative event, but with long-term positive consequences, as long as the event can be used as a springboard towards living a better life.

*I had never considered my mortality before. I'd had my neck lump for so long, I never thought it would threaten my life. Having thyroid cancer made me think carefully about the meaning of my life. The whole experience helped me change my values, which in turn helped me change the quality of my life. I used to focus on certain things, everyday things of normal life, then suddenly they had no meaning for me. People pursue their jobs, or money, but having cancer totally changed my values, and these things were no longer important for me. I'm now more focused on my family, on my community, on being more connected with people.*

## Sources of support

How we deal with these challenges is a personal thing, and what works for one person may not be the best answer for the next person. If things are looking bleak and you are finding things difficult to cope with, it's important that you seek the help and support that you need.

*You can't make life easy for everyone. Sometimes life is s\*\*t. There is certain stuff that you have to deal with, but with the right support it's not so hard.*

There are lots of potential sources of support, from your partner, or other family members, friends, colleagues, and neighbors. Then there are the professional groups – your family doctor who may be able to point you in the right direction - perhaps a clinical psychologist or trained counselor. There are also patient support groups – both those involving real people in the same room, and also the on-line support groups and chat rooms. Even if you have been a robust, resilient, bulletproof rock of a person all your life, it doesn't mean that you will never reach a breaking point, or that there is no situation that might be even a little difficult for you. Even the very best athletes, those that are naturally better than the rest of us, have their breaking point. None of us are immune from ever experiencing something for which we need the help of others. If you think you might be getting to that point, then ask for help, particularly if you have never needed to ask for help before. It will almost certainly help (and if it doesn't then ask someone else!) and is an important step towards you making the very best of whatever situation you find yourself in.

*"A man's pride can be his downfall, and he needs to learn when to turn to others for support and guidance"*

Bear Grylls

## Chapter 12 - Medullary thyroid cancer

Medullary thyroid cancer is an unusual type of thyroid cancer, which is quite different from the more common papillary and follicular types. That's why it gets its own chapter. The main difference is that medullary thyroid cancer (often known as MTC) does not develop from the thyroid cells that take up iodine and make thyroid hormone. Instead MTC develops from cells that just happen to be located within the thyroid, but have nothing to do with thyroid hormone production. The cells that MTC develop from are called C cells, and they often secrete a hormone called calcitonin. Calcitonin doesn't usually do very much, but in our distant evolutionary past it probably had something to do with controlling calcium levels in the blood. If calcitonin levels are very high, they can cause symptoms such as gut upset and diarrhea. Because MTC doesn't have anything to do with thyroid hormones, that means that it doesn't have the revolving doors on each cell to take up iodine, and so radioiodine is not useful in treating MTC.

Another important difference between MTC and most other thyroid cancers is that MTC can sometimes be hereditary (i.e. can be passed down through the generations) and it can sometimes be part of a wider syndrome that has other things that go along with it. The most common of the wider syndromes that MTC can be a part of is called Multiple Endocrine Neoplasia type 2, which can include other features such as parathyroid tumors (which cause high calcium levels), and tumors called phaeochromocytomas (usually located in the adrenal gland and can secrete adrenaline). This booklet is not the best place for an in-depth discussion of the many complex issues of MTC that might be inheritable. The more important thing to keep in mind is that the older you are when you develop MTC, the less likely it is to be of the hereditary type. If on the other hand you develop it at a relatively young age, and there is a family history of MTC or other tumors that secrete hormones, then it is more likely that you have a hereditary type of MTC. There are now genetic experts who can advise what best to do, including whether you might benefit from gene testing.

MTC is usually picked up either as part of family screening of relatives of someone known to have a familial form of MTC, or else it's picked up like other thyroid cancers (either as a lump that is felt, or one that is picked up on a scan done for something else). Occasionally a patient has bowel symptoms, and after all the usual causes have been investigated, someone thinks of the very rare cause of undiagnosed diarrhea – MTC – and then the calcitonin is measured and found to be very high, and then the search for the source of the calcitonin begins, usually with a scan of the thyroid and neck.

Once the MTC is found, the best form of treatment is surgical. Ideally the original tumor and thyroid is fully removed. If the MTC has spread to lymph nodes in the neck, then as many of these as can be reasonably removed should be taken out, to try to get the total volume of MTC cells remaining to be as small as possible. Having the calcitonin measured before surgery, and a number of weeks after surgery can give a rough idea what proportion of MTC cells have been removed. Sometimes the MTC has spread to other areas of the body other than the lymph nodes in the neck. If that it is the case then the location and size of these tumor deposits can help when deciding what best to do, but these are obviously complex and individualized discussions and decisions that would need to be made in conjunction with the various specialists with expertise in the area (thyroid physician, surgeon, oncologist, etc.). For those patients with very high calcitonin levels there are certain medications that can be used to help control the diarrhea.

Once the initial surgery has been performed, and things have moved into the follow-up phase, probably the most helpful tool for providing an idea of how things are going is the calcitonin level. MTC can behave in a wide variety of ways. For some it is a very slow-growing tumor that was probably present for many years before diagnosis, and what MTC cells that remain after surgery continue to grow very slowly and may never cause problems. For others it is a much more aggressive disease, with the cells growing fast and causing problems that may be very difficult, or impossible, to fully control, and the emphasis becomes control of symptoms. One thing that helps separate the slow-growing ones from the fast-growing ones is the calcitonin levels, or more specifically the rate of rise of the calcitonin levels. The time it takes for the calcitonin to double (unimaginatively called the calcitonin doubling time) is a good guide. Generally speaking the longer the calcitonin doubling time, the better. If the calcitonin doubling time is longer than 18 months, then it's more likely to be a slow-growing MTC, with a relatively good outcome, whereas if the calcitonin doubling time is shorter, particularly if it is less than 6 months, then it's more likely to be a faster-growing MTC. For those with the faster growing MTCs, there are a range of possible treatment options, including additional surgery or radiotherapy, and even inclusion in to a clinical trial of new medications. Again, the pros and cons of these options, and which and whether they are best for you, need to be carefully discussed with your specialists.

One practical point worth noting is that for calcitonin levels to be reliable, the blood sample often has to be handled carefully (it needs to be put on ice, and to get to the laboratory quickly), so make sure the people who take your calcitonin blood test are familiar with the process. It's a rare test and they may not do it often, and we often have patients who need to give a second sample because the first was not properly handled.

**Dealing with MTC**

MTC can be difficult to deal with. It presents a number of different challenges, which can be hard to get your head around. For those who have small tumors that have probably been completely removed at the initial surgery and the chances of it having spread elsewhere are small, they are likely to do well, with a good proportion having been genuinely cured by the surgery. There is still the angst of having to have check-ups for years, probably for life, with examinations, calcitonin measurements, etc. Even when the news from these follow-up appointments is usually good, that doesn't mean that there isn't the burden of worry and anxiety that goes along with such an experience. The trick is to try to minimize the total amount of time spent worrying and to reduce the degree of worry – quite how that is best achieved is often individual. Some genuinely aren't worriers, and take it as it comes, reassured by the knowledge that the chances of a good outcome are high, and if the news is not so good they will deal with that, and the various options, at the time. There are others whom are able to take an active choice not to worry until a certain date prior to clinic. At the other extreme there are those that are a wreck for weeks or months prior to their appointment, and every symptom of normal living is closely analyzed to see if it might represent a recurrence of MTC. In that situation the MTC is clearly detracting more from that person's quality of life than it should. If the focus is to get the most out of every day, then allowing MTC to impact negatively on many of those days is clearly not contributing to better living. If a mind-shift change towards living in the moment, and valuing the important things in life can be easily achieved, then there may not be the need to get expert help, but chances are that if you have been the type of person with tendencies towards anxiety, particularly health-related anxiety, then you will need to seek out those that can help. This may be clinical psychologist, skilled counselor, group help, etc., perhaps best guided by your own family doctor.

For those that are likely to have some MTC cells left after surgery – perhaps those with known spread to multiple lymph nodes, then coming to terms with a diagnosis of cancer that has already spread can be a huge challenge. With MTC there is the period after surgery, perhaps up to 2 years, where the calcitonin is checked every 6 months to see how any remaining cells are behaving. The range of outcomes is very wide, with some MTC tumors doing very little, growing very slowly and being unlikely to have any significant effect on long-term outlook. At the other extreme some MTC cells are quite abnormal and grow fast and may well require further treatment and even then could well affect that person's quality of life and be life-limiting. Facing such uncertainty is tough, sometimes really tough. There's no quick easy answer as to how best you should deal with this. However, coming back to some of the strategies mentioned earlier in this book might help;

1) Involve others (family, friends, healthcare professionals, etc.).

2) Try to take one day at a time, and then break things down further to one part of a day at a time, and bring the focus back to the present, the now, rather than the distant future.

3) Try to bring yourself more towards likely outcomes, rather than catastrophising to the worst (but very unlikely outcome).

4) If you identify an obstacle, try to think of what options there are for getting past that obstacle, put the best plan in place you can, and so reduce the power that obstacle has for negativity.

5) Be mindful of the stages of grief reactions, go with it, and do whatever helps to get you towards a point of acceptance.

6) If things aren't going well – seek whatever help you need – other books or internet resources, support groups, healthcare professionals, etc.

When the range of possible outcomes is very wide, there are too many possibilities to properly consider. Even if it was possible to properly consider them all, it would waste a lot of time and energy that could instead have been used to do more important and enjoyable things. When the outcome range is very wide, it's better to try to focus more on the present, if you can. However, once your calcitonin doubling time becomes clearer, then at least you can start narrowing down the range of likely outcomes. Even if it's not what you were hoping for, it can at least help you with planning. It can be a spring board to help you actually identify the things that are important to you, and from there help you draw up a plan of how best you can achieve as many of those important things as you can, as often as you can. You might be able to look back and see how much time you wasted in the past, and make an active choice to in the future (however long or short that might be) to spend as much time as you can on the things and people that you value the most.

## Family matters

An added dimension with MTC is the hereditary or familial aspect. There is the initial issue of whether your MTC is one that you may have inherited from one of your parents. Usually the inheritance is autosomal dominant which means that if a parent has it, then the chance of each of their children having it is 50%. Genetics is always more complicated than it first appears, and there are exceptions to most rules. MTC is often a new mutation which means that even though there may be no history of MTC in the parents of someone affected, the new mutation could be passed down to subsequent generations. Many MTCs are sporadic, which means that it has not been inherited from a parent, and cannot be passed on to a child. The older a person is when they get MTC, the more likely it is to be sporadic, and therefore of no direct consequence to family members. However, for those where the MTC may have been inherited and/or could be passed on, there is this additional issue of direct implications for family members. It's hard enough to deal with your own diagnosis, without having to consider that other family members may be similarly affected, or that you may have passed it on to your kids. This is exactly the situation I found myself in with my cardiac condition, which can be passed on to subsequent generations. This was horrible, and whilst I was in a psychological spin about my own diagnosis and uncertain future, the possibility that I may have given it to my young children was gut-wrenchingly awful. However, I received expert help and the key here was to actively nip those feelings of guilt in the bud. We are all dealt a genetic hand of cards at birth, and as parents we not only contribute 50/50 to those cards of our kids (which we have no control over), but we are also responsible for the environment in which they are nurtured (which we have much more control over). In the huge hand of genetic cards that we have given to our children, most of them will be top quality cards from which they have and will continue to benefit from. In amongst them will be the odd genetic dud, but particularly if we had no knowledge that there were some duds in our pack, there is no way you could know about them or control which were dealt. You cannot feel guilty about something that you had no knowledge or control over. As a parent you can have control over the environment in which you nurture your kids – the time you spend with them, the love and care you provide. If you concentrate on being the best parent you can be, getting the most out of every moment you have with them, then this is the positive way to channel any guilty or negativity you may have felt about them happening to pick up some of your dud genetic cards. Don't beat yourself up about what has happened in the past, but instead concentrate on making each present and future moment as good as it can be.

On a practical note, if you are found to have a familial form of MTC, then at least that means that your family can be tested for the same gene, and for those family members that are positive, then they can get treatment early (such as surgical thyroidectomy to catch MTC early, or even before it has developed), and so their outcome is likely to be better than if their MTC had only shown itself much further down the track.

So whilst MTC is quite different from other more common types of thyroid cancer, it shares many characteristics. These include the initial diagnosis being massively unwelcome, that the future will initially be very uncertain, but with time the likely range of outcomes will become clearer. These outcomes could well be different from what you had expected out of life, but this presents an opportunity to focus on the important stuff, to live in the present, and to make you live better in whatever amount of time you have.

# Chapter 13 - Anaplastic thyroid cancer

Being honest, anaplastic thyroid cancer is not something I know very much about, not only because it is rare, but also because endocrinologists aren't often involved in the care of patients with this type of tumor. Anaplastic thyroid cancer makes up less than 1% of all thyroid cancers, and it usually affects those aged over 65 years. It typically shows itself as a firm, fairly fast-growing, lump in the neck, which leads to an FNA from which decisions about what best to do and who best to do it can be made. There is usually involvement of a surgeon, and cancer doctors (oncologists). The reality of anaplastic thyroid cancer is that it is usually fast-growing, aggressive and very difficult to control. Some people benefit from having surgery to remove as much of it as possible, but it's almost never possible to remove it all as the tumor has often already spread locally into surrounding tissues in the neck. Anaplastic thyroid cancer doesn't respond to radioiodine. Some patients benefit from radiotherapy, delivered as an external beam of radiotherapy (rather than radioiodine which delivers the radioactivity from the inside of the thyroid cells). This external beam radiotherapy is sometimes combined with chemotherapy, but anaplastic thyroid cancer is well known for being fairly resistant to such treatment with overall results being far below what everyone involved would want.

Anaplastic thyroid cancer is one of those-life changing diagnoses. The likely outcome is that it will have a major effect on a person's quality of life, and will likely have a similar effect on quantity of life. It will almost certainly be life-limiting, unless it affects someone who is already very unwell from other medical problems. Coping with the diagnosis has to consider the backdrop of the typical life expectancy of anaplastic thyroid cancer being around 5 months, with about 1 in 5 people being alive 1 year after their diagnosis. There are of course exceptions, with some people succumbing very quickly, whereas a few can survive for 5 years or more. The likely outcome is somewhere in the middle, usually months rather than weeks or years.

In the setting of anaplastic thyroid cancer, where quantity of life is very likely to be very limited, then the priority is to maximize the quality of every remaining day. Whilst some of the themes of this book are still relevant for anaplastic thyroid cancer, the timeline is such that there is no time to waste, and things need to be done quickly if you want to be sure that they will happen. From a medical perspective the Palliative Care Team is usually involved. They are usually fantastic at looking at your symptoms and coming up with effective and imaginative ways of controlling those symptoms, such that you are more able to do the things that you want to do, in the maximum comfort. They have seen it all before and can talk things through with you so that you are informed and prepared for each of the stages, knowing that they are there to help you all the way.

A detailed discussion about the management of anaplastic thyroid cancer is outside of the scope of a short book like this. More importantly the discussions that need to happen depend on your individual circumstances of not only your tumor and how advanced it is, but in the context of you, your family, what other medical issues you may have, what medical services are available, what your priorities are, and how you want to manage things. Getting a quick diagnosis, and developing a prompt but carefully thought-out management plan is crucial, involving all the necessary specialists (but no more than necessary) and involving palliative care as soon as you may need their help. Once the plan is in place, this can allow you some time to focus on doing what needs to be done, saying what needs to be said, and getting the most out of every remaining day.

*"The end of a melody is not its goal: but nonetheless, had the melody not reached its end it would not have reached its goal either."*

Friedrich Nietzsche

# Chapter 14 - Thyroid hormone replacement in thyroid cancer

Thyroid hormones are crucial for life. If you go without them for too long, things do not go well. Thyroid hormones are like the accelerator on your car. If thyroid hormone levels are high, it's like putting the foot down. You speed up, your engine revs up and you get hot. You burn off fuel, and eventually you burn out. If your thyroid hormone levels are too low, it like putting the brakes on – you slow down, you get lethargic, you feel the cold, and eventually grind to a halt.

The key is of course to get the levels right. There are well-known ranges that thyroid hormones should remain within, for the normal, healthy population. An individual tends to run a narrower range of fluctuation compared to this fairly wide population normal range. With very rare exceptions, if you can keep your thyroid hormone levels in the population normal range, you are extremely unlikely to experience symptoms related to your thyroid hormone levels.

The 3 key thyroid hormones are TSH (thyroid stimulation hormone), T4 and T3. T4 is the main thyroid hormone released by the thyroid gland into the bloodstream, and levels in the blood fluctuate relatively slowly. T4 goes to pretty much every cell in the body, where it does its thing, keeping the body's metabolic engine purring along at the right speed. Once T4 gets inside the cells of the body, it gets converted to T3 which is the main active thyroid hormone at the cellular level.

In contrast, TSH comes from the pituitary gland and stimulates the thyroid to produce thyroid hormones (T3 and T4) and release them into the bloodstream. Importantly, TSH is also like fertilizer for the thyroid, helping the thyroid cells to survive and grow. This is a good thing in the normal situation, but can be a bad thing in thyroid cancer. If someone has had surgery for thyroid cancer and their thyroid has been removed, they need thyroid hormone replacement in the form of tablets, in order to keep their metabolic engine healthy. If there are any thyroid cancer cells left in the body, perhaps some small deposits in some lymph nodes, we obviously don't want to do anything that might encourage them to grow. Instead the aim is for those thyroid cancer cells to remain dormant, and not to cause any future problems. Therefore we don't want to bathe them in TSH fertilizer, but instead have the TSH level low. This is done by giving a dose of thyroid hormone replacement that is marginally higher than is required, so that the pituitary is satisfied that there is plenty of thyroid hormone around, and so it doesn't need to release TSH. The aim is for T4 and T3 levels to be close to the upper limit of normal, with a TSH that is consequently low. We don't want the T4 and T3 to be too high such that they cause symptoms of hyperthyroidism, and so sometimes some compromises need to be made.

Usually after surgery for thyroid cancer the aim is to keep the TSH low for at least a few years so there is time to see how the thyroid cancer is behaving. If there are no signs of any recurrence then the need to keep the TSH low diminishes (if there are no thyroid cancer cells remaining, then there is no need to try to keep them dormant), and the thyroid hormone replacement dose may be reduced, aiming for TSH levels in the lower half of the normal range. The downside of having a low TSH for some years is that it can have a modest thinning effect on your bones which could contribute to future osteoporosis, causing weak bones that are prone to fracture. Also a low TSH for years can increase the chance of developing a heart rhythm called atrial fibrillation. This is quite common in later years, even without a low TSH, but a low TSH makes it more likely to occur. If it does occur it can make the heart less effective as a pump, so reducing exercise capacity. Also the erratic flow of blood through the heart can allow small blood clots to form, which can then travel in the bloodstream, and if they lodge in an artery in the brain they can block blood flow and cause a stroke. People in atrial fibrillation are often on blood thinners (such as warfarin or dabigatran) to reduce the chance of stroke. Whilst this is quite effective, it does increase the risk of bleeding, which causes its own problems. The take home message is that it's best to avoid atrial fibrillation if possible.

Therefore if you need your TSH suppressed in order to improve the outcome from your thyroid cancer, then that's all good, and the modest longer term risks of thin bones and atrial fibrillation are trumped by the positive effect of low TSH at helping keep your thyroid cancer under control. However if your thyroid cancer is of low risk of causing you future trouble, and there's no signs of recurrence, then the balance of net benefit swings away from having a long term low TSH, towards having a normal TSH that returns your bones and risk of atrial fibrillation back to normal.

One key practical point is that if ever someone wants to change your thyroid hormone replacement dose, then you need to make sure that they know of your previous thyroid cancer and know what your specialist wants your TSH to be. Otherwise it's very easy for someone to see your thyroid hormone results, and mistake them for unintentional over-replacement of thyroid hormone, and drop the dose back to 'normal', when in fact it is *intentional* slight over-replacement of thyroid hormone to help manage your thyroid cancer.

**Taking thyroid hormone replacement**

I don't know anyone that wants to be taking tablets. Having to take medication can be a daily reminder that our health is not as perfect as it once was or as we would like it to be. It takes some adjustment, but I'd suggest it is wasted emotion and energy to be overly upset about being on medication. If you do feel upset about being on medication, sufficiently upset that a neutral observer might think you were overly upset, then I'd encourage you to consider the current options. If you've had your thyroid removed, then if you don't take thyroid hormone replacement then you will feel increasingly unwell and will eventually die from lack of thyroid hormone. If you do take them, you should feel physically the same from a thyroid hormone perspective as you did before you required thyroid hormone replacement. For the neutral observer the best option is clear.

What some people do (including what I did, at least for a while) is instead of comparing current options, they compare their current situation to their previous situation. The comparison then becomes between taking tablets now and feeling ok (but upset at having to take tablets), compared to in the past when I felt well and didn't need to take tablets. This is an unhelpful comparison, which doesn't contribute towards you getting the most out of today and future days. It's backward-looking and unconstructive, yet I think it is a natural thought process, at least for a while, as you come to terms with your new reality. It's perhaps part of a mini-grieving process, that needs some time to work itself through. The aim is to get through that process before too long, before too much unnecessary time and emotion is expended, to get to the point of acceptance of that fact that taking tablets today is a welcomed outcome. In previous times, when there was no sophisticated surgery or other treatments for thyroid cancer, then you could well have been dead before your current age. However, now there are the treatments and medications available that can offer you a far better outlook, and appreciating this makes the treatments and medication much easier to take.

Once you have (hopefully) got to the point of acceptance regarding the need for medications, in this case thyroid hormone replacement, there are some practical issues to consider. Thyroid hormone preparations are not drugs that interfere with or stimulate the body's thyroid hormone manufacture processes, they are simply the same stuff that your thyroid previously made (T4). The body doesn't care where it's come from (your own thyroid or from a swallowed tablet), just so long as the level of T4 in the bloodstream is OK. The thyroid gland usually makes some T3 as well as T4, and thyroid hormone replacement is usually just T4, but given that the body converts T4 into T3, then there is no need for additional T3 replacement. There is a sometimes quite a debate about whether someone should also have T3 replacement. I don't intend to get into that debate, other than to say that I haven't yet seen anyone whom appeared to really need T3 supplements (they would have to be unable to convert T4 to T3 for them to actually need T3 replacement, and this would have been the case prior to their thyroid cancer), but a small minority of patients report feeling better on T3. I'm not sure if this is a placebo effect (which is probably the most common reason for a positive effect from taking T3, which wears off with time), or whether there is a physiological explanation, but almost always the effect wears off with time. I'd strongly recommend you stick to just common or garden T4, as it almost always does the job, with less peaks and troughs in thyroid hormone levels. If it's not working, despite the desired blood hormone levels, then that's the time to discuss it with your specialist.

When taking T4 there are a few things to bear in mind. T4 tablets (often known as thyroxine) can bind to things that are in the gut at the same time, such as calcium and iron. If the T4 binds to these elements, then the T4 can't get fully absorbed and so some of the T4 is lost in the faeces. Therefore if you are having fluctuating thyroid hormone levels it may be because there are other things in the gut at the same time. If this is the case taking the T4 at a different time to food or calcium or iron tablets can fix the problem. Also the half-life of T4 is quite long, about 1 week. The half-life of T4 is the amount of time it takes for your blood levels of T4 to drop by half, after stopping taking the T4. This means that T4 levels don't tend to change quickly, or fluctuate much from day to day. Therefore if you forget a day's T4, it's fine to catch up the following day by taking twice the dose on that day.

From seeing hundreds of patients on thyroid hormone replacement I can count on one hand the number of people who have never missed a dose. It's human to err, and I think for most humans it's impossible to remember it every day. What is most effective in the situation of fluctuating thyroid hormone levels possibly due to variable intake, is to buy a dosette box (from your pharmacy or $2 shop), that has a compartment for each day of the week. On a Sunday evening, load-up each of the day's compartment with the correct dose of T4. Then take it each day. If you find that you've forgotten a day then you'll see it in the box. As soon as you realize you've missed a day (or days!), then on that day catch-up all the forgotten doses, so that by the end of the week you can be sure that your total weekly intake has been constant. In this setting it's so much easier for your doctor to adjust the dose and get your TSH exactly where it should be.

Because of the long half-life of thyroxine, it's best to leave 4 to 6 weeks between making adjustments to the thyroid hormone dose, so that your blood levels have reached a steady state, from which further dose adjustments can be estimated.

If the thyroid hormone levels are still fluctuating despite the above steps, the next thing to consider is whether there may be an absorption issue due to some bowel problem, such as coeliac disease, and further investigations into these possibilities may be required.

Of course, everyone is different, and it may take some time and adjustments before you are fully happy taking thyroxine, and the blood levels are where they need to be. But in the long run, this can be put in the basket of things too small to waste time worrying about. Once it's sorted, you can get on with getting the most out of each day.

*"We have won the time lottery of the last 4 billion years."*

Stefan Molyneux

# Chapter 15 - Closing thoughts

Life is often not easy. Huge challenges may appear when we least expect them and when we are least able to deal with them. Life deals each of us a hand of cards, plus we pick up a few along the way. It's perhaps not so much the cards we have, but how we play them, that determines the outcome, and the amount of enjoyment we have along the way. If life was easy, it would arguably be less rewarding. The greatest satisfaction can come from overcoming life's obstacles. However, sometimes an obstacle appears too big to be climbed over alone, and that's when we need to seek all the support we can get, to call in all the favors, and together get to the other side, ready for the next hurdle, and ready to help someone else if they need your support for their hurdle.

This book can never answer all the questions that relate to thyroid cancer, but instead is aimed to just be a beginner's guide. Written from my perspective of having been on both sides of the patient / doctor relationship, I felt the need to begin to address some of the more psychological aspects that go along with such a medical problem as thyroid cancer. However I'm fully aware that trying to begin to deal with all the psychological stuff, in my amateurish way, may be unnecessary for many, and only scratching the surface for others. I'm hoping that it will help at least some, if only to identify that they need more expert help than this book can provide.

I'm also hoping that your diagnosis of thyroid cancer can be used as a catalyst for positive change. Whilst that may seem odd, and unlikely at first, I'm hoping that with whatever time that can be provided by the good care of your thyroid cancer, that this time can be used in the best possible way. I hope that from here on you can overcome your fears, and find fulfillment, so that you can live better with thyroid cancer than you ever did before.

*"Don't cry because it's over,
smile because it happened."*

- Dr Seuss

## Thanks

I'd like to thank the patients who allowed me to interview them and were willing to share their own experiences with me and with the wider thyroid cancer community. I've not included their names in this book, and I've changed the names for the various quotes we've used in the website, but they know who they are!

I'd also like to thank the patients who took the time to read earlier drafts of this book (particularly Graeme, Helen and Karen). Their generous time and feedback has really helped make this book so much better than it was.

Thanks also to Dr David Cole, Dr Sorcha Nic Giolla, Hilary Totty and Chris Bailey for their editorial help and general encouragement.

I'm grateful to so many other people I couldn't possibly list them all, but I'd like to mention the staff at Christchurch Hospital (including Dr Paul Bridgman, Cardiologist and Mr Harsh Singh, Cardiothoracic Surgeon), the patients I have met, my colleagues, my friends and my family – they all help keep me truly alive.

www.thyroidcancer.support

Printed in Great Britain
by Amazon